Once a Month

"This book was written with the aim of spreading the news to mankind that the once-a-month miseries of countless women can be, and are being, successfully relieved and treated. At the same time it was hoped that it would help men to understand and appreciate the menstrual problems of women and become partners in helping them through those difficult days. That you are reading this brings hope that the aim will be achieved."

From the Book

"ONCE A MONTH is the single most important book I have ever read. It certainly saved my sanity and quite possibly my life. You can't know how grateful I am to you—and the gratitude is profoundly shared by my husband and our son."

M.T.I., Waynesburg, Pa.

About the Author

Katharina Dalton was born in England, in 1916. Her early training was as a chiropodist at the London Foot Hospital, where she wrote *Essentials of Chiropody*, now a basic textbook. Widowed during the war, she started medical training at the Royal Free Hospital, worked in the evenings, remarried and had three children. In 1948 she qualified as an MD and entered general practice. Her personal experiences and her interest in the menstrual cycle resulted in 1953 in the first paper in British medical literature on the premenstrual syndrome, written in collaboration with Dr. Raymond Greene.

Dr. Dalton is now an acknowledged authority on the part played by menstrual dysfunctions in confused and criminal behavior, accidents, drug abuse and morbidity. Her work on premenstrual syndrome and its treatment with progesterone therapy is applied in factories, schools, prisons, shops and hospitals, and she has received numerous awards for her research. She lectures extensively and has appeared on television in Europe and the U.S., has a consultant practice based in London's famous Harley Street and holds a premenstrual clinic attended by medical students at the University College Hospital. In 1971 she became the first woman President of the General Practice section of the Royal Society of Medicine. She was an expert witness in two cases of murder in which premenstrual syndrome was accepted as a factor causing diminished responsibility, thus making legal history in Britain.

Her books and publications include *The Premenstrual Syndrome* (1964), *The Menstrual Cycle* (1970), *The Premenstrual Syndrome and Progesterone Therapy* (1977), and *Depression after Childbirth* (1980), which are widely used in the medical profession. Through her work, research and writing she is advancing medical and lay knowledge of menstrual problems and their effects, and bringing discussion of them out into the open so that a great deal of unnecessary female suffering and insecurity may be overcome once and for all.

Once a Month

KATHARINA DALTON, M.D.

Hunter House

Grateful acknowledgment is given the following for permission to reprint copyrighted material:

"The Importance of Diagnosing Premenstrual Syndrome" from *Health Visitor*, 1982
"Legal Implications of PMS" from *World Medicine*, 1982

First published in Great Britain by Fontana Paperbacks 1978

© Katharina Dalton 1979, 1983

First U.S. edition published in 1979 by Hunter House Inc. Publishers

Second (revised) U.S. edition published in 1983 by
Hunter House Inc. Publishers
P.O. Box 1302
Claremont, CA 91711

ISBN 0-89793-030-4

Cover design by Qalagraphia
Set in 11 on 12 point Goudy Old Style by Freedmen's Organization, Los Angeles, CA
Printed and bound in the USA

Contents

Contents *(Continued)*

List of Figures

List of Figures *(continued)*

Preface to Second Edition

In 1954 speaking to the General Practice Section of the Royal Society of Medicine, I ended my paper with the words:

> "The cost of progesterone therapy is high, but when this is weighed against the price in terms of human misery, suffering and injustice, it is seen as a justifiable expense opening up a new vista of Medicine."

That vista is still opening up and during the last few years considerable progress has been made in the appreciation and understanding of menstrual problems and their treatment by the caring professions and also by the general public.

At the symposium on Premenstrual Syndrome at the International Congress of Psychosomatic Obstetrics and Gynecology held in Berlin in September 1980, it was agreed that the premenstrual syndrome was a hormonal disease, therefore it was more suited for study by international meetings of endocrinologists rather than by psychologists. Of course there will always be those who disagree and suggest other approaches, which is as it should be, provided they are talking about the same diagnosed disease and have tried the same treatments comparing them with other treatments to find the most successful.

New issues have emerged, such as the legal implications and the feminist movement. The premenstrual syndrome should not be a feminist issue. It is a hormonal disease, which deserves sympathy and understanding and requires to be diagnosed and treated.

This edition has been widely revised in the light of the findings of the past four years and includes a new Appendix on "Legal Implications." It is as up-to-date as it is possible to be, in the hope that the disease will be more commonly recognized, correctly diagnosed and properly treated.

Dr. Katharina Dalton

London, 1983.

Preface to
First Edition

This book is dedicated to the thousands of women who have confided in me the most personal and intimate details of their lives and from whom I have learned so much.

I am deeply grateful for the help received from all my family. To Drs. Maureen and Michael Dalton who have been my most severe critics; to Mrs. Anita Dalton and Mrs. Wendy Holton who have patiently typed, corrected and re-typed the manuscript before it was ready for submission to the publishers; to my niece, Mrs. Sherryl Machray for the artwork; to Mrs. Sharlynn Orr who has kindly adapted my work for America; and most of all to my long-suffering husband, Rev. Tom Dalton for his invaluable ghost-writing of the entire book.

Finally, my acknowledgement to David Duff and Tandem Press for the excerpt from *Albert & Victoria*, and the Journal of the Royal College of General Practitioners for permission to reproduce Figure 11.

Katharina Dalton

1978

Introduction

Once-a-month, with monotonous regularity, chaos is inflicted on American homes as premenstrual tension and other menstrual problems recur time and time again with demoralizing repetition. This book explains how these menstrual problems can be completely relieved with the proper treatment, just as the pains of childbirth are today universally treated with pain-relievers and anesthetics.

It has also been written to help men to understand the capricious and temperamental changes of women, so that the image of woman as uncertain, fickle, changeable, moody and hard to please may go, to be replaced with the recognition that all these features can be understood in terms of the ever-changing ebb and flow of her menstrual hormones.

It was as long ago as 1948 that I came across my first case of premenstrual asthma, which responded successfully to treatment with progesterone. Before a month had passed a further case of asthma, two of epilepsy and one of migraine had been found, all related to menstruation. However, for the premenstrual syndrome to be properly appreciated it must be recognized in all its full variety. Following a recent television documentary on the subject which showed only four presentations – an alcoholic, a baby-batterer, a husband-beater and a neurotic – the hospital's postbag was filled with letters which suggested that the program had been an eye-opener to many viewers, whose letters contained such comments as:

"It was such a relief to know that so many other women experience the very real and deep feelings of anger, hatred and depression that I feel at period times."

"I'm just like that woman."

"I never told anyone because I thought they would never believe me."

It is hoped this book will open many more eyes for it is estimated that there are in America today over 5½ million women with incapacitating monthly problems which can and should be eased.

The first step is to bring the subject out into the open, and not to sweep it under the carpet. Menstruation should be a subject that can be discussed as openly as sex; anywhere, by anybody, not merely in the bedroom or doctor's office. We still suffer from the utterly Victorian attitude in which heroines in novels never menstruate. If women themselves do not yet associate the changes in their body and psyche with the changes in menstrual hormones, how can one hope that men will be able to understand them? After all, men don't even experience it. There must be a general recognition of the physical and psychological changes in a woman which occur like a flash of lightning before menstruation, and which are not due to personality inadequacies.

While accepting that fatalities from the premenstrual syndrome or period pains are rare and the suffering is short-lived, ending with menstruation, nevertheless the suffering, unhappiness and social consequences of it are without limitation.

One gynecologist ranks the premenstrual syndrome as the commonest cause of marital breakdown. In a general practice survey in England 75% of a sample of 521 women complained of at least one premenstrual symptom. In Britain the attempted suicide rate shows that there is a seven-fold increase in the second half of the menstrual cycle compared with the pre-ovulatory half. Shoplifting is thirty times commoner in the second half of the cycle. Of 132 women who were currently under the care of the Premenstrual Syndrome Clinic at University College Hospital, London, during December 1977, 37% had a previous mental hospital admission; 34% had attempted suicide or homicide; 9% had alcoholic bouts; 6% were referred because of actual child abuse and a further 4% sought treatment because of a fear of their injuries to their children becoming public knowledge; 6% had a history of criminal behavior, such as smashing the windows of the Social Services headquarters, assaulting police or neighbors; 7% had premenstrual epilepsy and 5% had premenstrual asthma.

These are no trivialities but are of vital concern to the patient, her family, society, and maybe even a nation. This is shown in the following extract from *Albert & Victoria*, David Duff's book on the married life of Queen Victoria (London: Muller, 1972):

> "One of the reasons why Victoria continued to bear children was her belief that, by doing so, she kept her grip on Albert . . . When she was pregnant he was always kind, thoughtful, attentive of her every wish. Here was a problem that he could understand, a train of events to which he could attend. But he knew nothing of the imponderable in women. He was completely inexperienced. He did not appreciate the unreasoned emotions which surged like a maelstrom in Victoria's brain. Albert's answer to all the problems of life was to exercise reason . . . When Victoria began throwing things and screaming her accusations into his face, he would retire to write a paper on the cause of the outburst. She would then receive a letter beginning "Dear Child" and containing simple ingredients for an antidote to emotion.

This did not help matters. Albert soon learned that any action that he took at such times was wrong. Answering back led to faster, louder vituperation. Remaining quiet was classified as insulting. Retiring behind a locked door eventually led to an attack upon its panels by royal fists. . . . Even (Lord) Melbourne, a past master at dealing with women, had on one occasion quavered and feared to sit down as the fire blazed in the eyes of the eighteen-year-old queen. A cabinet minister was known to fly from her presence, too frightened to follow the rule of withdrawal. Thus Albert looked forward to the period of pregnancy – it gave emotion a reason."

The premenstrual syndrome knows no geographical, social, racial or economic boundaries; its sufferings and trage- dies are spread evenly throughout our society. For many it is sufficient reassurance to know that other normal women also experience the same monthly feelings, while the knowl- edge that there is a satisfactory answer provides them with hope for the future.

1

The Curse of Eve

Once a month women are reminded that their reproductive system is still in the process of evolution. But it is no good waiting another two or three million years for Mother Nature to iron out the flaws. In the short term it is better to try to understand the way our body works, the problems with which the silent majority tries to cope and how best they can be helped.

The other natural functions of the body, such as growth, respiration, digestion and excretion go on day by day without pain. Indeed if pain is present it is abnormal, a cause for concern, and a thorough search is made to find and eradicate the disease. On the other hand the two natural feminine physiological processes, menstruation and childbirth, are seldom completely without pain. It is thought that less than one woman in five goes through her childbearing years without at some time suffering from period pain or premenstrual tension. It is now universally accepted (although it was not always so) that women experiencing pain during labor are deserving of relief with analgesics and anesthetics, and they even go into training for this one-day event with weekly relaxation classes. One hopes that the days of enlightenment are not too far off when treatment for the relief of period pains and premenstrual problems will be accepted as the natural right of every woman the world over.

Menstruation represents a failed pregnancy, and only

occurs if the woman is neither pregnant nor breastfeeding. It is therefore perhaps a cultural disease, which did not occur in primitive societies where women went from one pregnancy to another until the menopause was reached. With today's families limited to two children, normal women may expect at least three hundred menstruations before the end comes with the menopause.

Anne, 34 years, was brought to the doctor's office by the Catholic priest, because of a severe asthma attack which accompanied her last menstruation. She was asked if asthma had also accompanied her previous menstruation before this last one. She took a few minutes to think about it before admitting "I was only eighteen at the time and I can't really remember." She had fourteen children, and for the last 16 years had either been pregnant or breastfeeding.

Pain is not the only symptom associated with menstruation: there are also the psychological and bodily symptoms which come out of the blue once a month, usually just before menstruation, and come under the omnibus heading of the Premenstrual Syndrome. Examples include Barbara and Carol.

Barbara wrote:

"I have such drastic changes in personality before a period I think I am going mad. I cannot understand how I can feel so differently towards my children, one day loving and caring for them and the next day hateful and rough, so bad-tempered and smacking them for nothing. How guilty I feel when I see my own daughter, aged five, copying me and smacking her dolls."

Carol wrote:

"I have one fantastic week each month, but after ovulation my whole body changes, my breasts start to swell, I look five months pregnant with a swollen tummy, my chest is tight and I just can't breathe because of asthma, There is usually a migraine on the first day of menstruation."

Relief is possible for women with painful periods and also for those with premenstrual symptoms, like Barbara and Carol. However, first it is necessary for them to realize the association between their symptoms and menstruation, which means it depends either on the patient herself recognizing it, or her husband, mother or close friend, or her doctor. Once the problem is recognized, treatment is available, as will be seen in later chapters.

It has been said "Man is born to suffer, but woman is born to suffer more" and sometimes it seems that no efforts are being made to ease a woman's sufferings. Consider this list of excuses culled from recent letters:

"It's not fatal and doesn't last long"

"She'll get over it"

"Cool it, lady, you're neurotic"

"Things will be easier when you're married" . . . "or had children" . . . "or the children have grown up"

"Learn to live with it and take more exercise"

"Accept the symptoms – you're not going mad – and learn to relax"

"Only because you've not enough to do" (three children, all under school age)

"You're working too hard" (one child at school)

"You're only trying to jump on the bandwagon like 90% of other women"

And so the excuses go on with the adoption of an ostrich-like attitude to once-a-month problems and no efforts made to solve them.

There is nothing new about these menstrual problems, even Hippocrates, the father of medicine, blamed premenstrual tension on "the agitated blood of a woman seeking a way of escape from the womb." Primitive man found it difficult to understand how women could lose blood month by month, yet neither be ill nor die. Even today many men are amazed that women can accept the regular loss of blood so cheerfully, when they themselves panic each time their nose bleeds or they cut a finger. But it is only rarely that women complain of the blood itself; it is how they feel and look, and the pains they suffer, that worries them. When primitive tribes lived in isolation there might be only one menstruating woman present at any one time. It was natural then to endow her with supernatural powers, normally ascribed to their gods. These powers included her ability to stop hailstorms, whirlwinds and lightning if she went out into the open unclothed. Menstrual blood was also thought to be endowed with valuable properties, such as being able to extinguish fires, temper metals and fashion swords as well as protecting men against wounds in battle. A thread soaked in menstrual blood was considered a valuable treatment for epilepsy and headache (today we often find that once menstruation starts, the premenstrual epilepsy or headache is relieved).

Myths about menstruation are worldwide. In some parts the presence of a menstruating woman was believed to cause harm, being able to sour wines, blight crops, rust iron or bronze and turn copper green. She could cause cattle to abort, seeds to dry up, fruit on trees to die, bright mirrors to become dulled, the edge to be taken off sharpened metal, a hive of bees to perish, the strings of harps to break, clocks to stop and linen to turn black. Can one wonder that women in India went into *purdah* at these times?

During the Middle Ages it was believed that menstruation demonstrated the essential sinfulness and inferiority of women, who were therefore forbidden to attend church or take communion, a custom still observed in the Greek Orthodox Church today. For this reason also, Orthodox Jewish women are instructed to make themselves plain and unattractive during menstruation to avoid exciting their husbands sexually. Following menstruation, the woman is required to undergo a ritualistic cleansing by immersing herself three times in a "body of water."

In different countries there are many local customs associated with menstruation, which are concerned chiefly with the local industries and fear of their failure. In Indonesia, menstruating women may not enter tobacco fields or work in rice paddies. In Saigon they may not be employed in opium factories, lest the opium turn bitter. In France and Germany they were excluded from the wineries and breweries lest they turned wine or beer sour; and in the Canary Islands today women are not allowed in the grape-crushing area. In France, the presence of a menstruating woman during the boiling process in sugar refineries might turn the sugar black. Parsee women in India may not look at a fire lest their glance extinguish it. In Syria, if pickling is done by menstruating women it will cause the food to putrefy. In South Africa, menstruating women may not come into contact with cattle for fear the milk will turn sour. Until the last century in England it was believed that if menstruating women salted meat it would not keep.

The problems associated with menstruation are obviously not new, they represent the eternal mystery of women. What is new is the changing attitude of the medical profession which now contains a few doctors, far too few, who have interested themselves in these problems and have shown that they can be successfully treated, and treated without witchcraft. These doctors see this shamefully neglected subject of menstruation, with its complexity of symptoms which can change a woman from Jekyll to Hyde within minutes, as a challenge to be met.

THE MENSTRUAL CYCLE

Woman is born with two ovaries containing thousands of immature egg cells. Each month, in response to a message from the pituitary gland, one of the unripe egg cells develops inside a tiny microscopic ring of cells, which gradually increases to form a little balloon or cyst called the Graafian follicle. These cells of the ovary make the menstrual hormone, *estrogen*, about which we will be hearing much more later. When the little egg cell is fully developed, it appears as a blister on the surface of the ovary and under a further message from the pituitary gland it bursts and releases the mature egg cell. When this occurs it is known as *ovulation*. The egg cell makes its way down the fallopian tubes to the womb, a journey that takes about fourteen days. Meanwhile, the yellow scar tissue left behind when the blister bursts fills up with new cells which produce the second important menstrual hormone, *progesterone*. The progesterone acts on the lining of the womb to turn it into a soft spongy layer in which the fertilized egg cell can embed itself if a pregnancy occurs. During intercourse millions of male sperm are projected into the vagina and journey through the womb into the tube in an attempt to fertilize the egg cell so that conception will occur and pregnancy can begin. The fertilized egg passes into the womb and becomes embedded in the new soft lining where it develops into a baby.

However, if the egg cell has not been fertilized it passes out of the womb. About 14 days after ovulation the soft spongy lining of the womb, which is then not needed, disintegrates and is shed as menstrual blood or *menstruation.*

PHASES OF THE MENSTRUAL CYCLE

Menstrual cycles vary considerably in length in different women, so that ovulation does not necessarily occur precisely on day 14, but for the purpose of understanding the changes in the menstrual cycle it is convenient to divide it up into seven phases of four days each, which assumes the woman has a precise cycle of twenty-eight days. It will be noticed that in the seven phases there are no two phases which have the same levels of hormones circulating in the blood. (Figure 1)

The phases are:

Days 1– 4	*Menstruation* with rising estrogen levels
Days 5– 8	*Postmenstruum* with peak estrogen levels
Days 9–12	*Late postmenstruum* with falling estrogen levels
Days 13–16	*Ovulation* with low estrogen and peak levels of follicle stimulating hormones and luteinising hormones
Days 17–20	*Post-Ovulation* with rising estrogen and progesterone levels

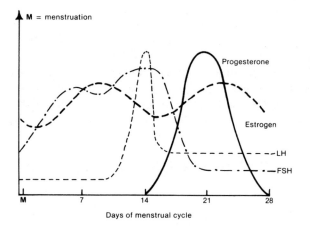

Figure 1   Menstrual hormone variations
during the menstrual cycle

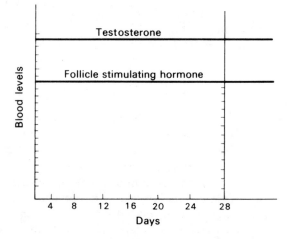

Figure 2   Male hormone levels during a month

Days 21–24   *Early premenstruum* with peak estrogen
              and progesterone levels
Days 25–28   *Premenstruum* with falling levels of estro-
              gen and progesterone

The first four days of menstruation and the last four days before menstruation are known as the *paramenstruum*. It is a useful term which is used in surveys, for these days occur regardless of the length of a woman's cycle. In long cycles the postmenstruum will be longer than eight days while short cycles will have a short postmenstruum. For comparison the daily levels of male hormones are steady day by day, as shown in Figure 2.

The attitudes of women to regular menstruation vary considerably. Some think of it as a sign of normality and an indication of good health. Others regard it as a sign of femininity with maternal attributes, or it may be just an assurance that the woman is not pregnant now but is fertile. Menopausal women see menstruation as a sign of their youthfulness to which they are so anxious to cling, whilst those who see menstruation as a once-a-month nuisance, to be tolerated as Mother Nature's wish, wonder why medical scientists have not given more thought to the abolition of the associated ailments and complaints.

A study of the words used throughout the world to describe menstruation is fascinating. In Jamaica, Nigeria, Egypt and Mexico words are used to imply a state of ill-health or pain, such as "being unwell" or "having the blues." In Yugoslavia, Mexico, Egypt and the Phillipines the menstrual bleeding is often personified as a "visitor," also in Britain it may be "the curse" or given the familiarity of an old friend like "Charlie" or "Archie." In Nigeria and Jamaica young girls are taught about "growing up" using the analogy of "Flowers and Bees" so that when menstruation occurs it is called "flowers." Women in Egypt and Korea often use terms associated with sanitary pads and bathing. In Indonesia the words used are associated with pollution or with purification. In the Phillipines the phrase "desire for abortion" is sometimes used when describing menstruation.

Psychologists object to the use of the word "curse" claiming that it conditions women to expect trouble with menstruation. On the other hand women have as many menstrual problems in Nigeria and Jamaica where the word "flowers" is used. There is no doubt that psychological factors do play a part in menstrual problems, but this is only secondary to the hormonal effects.

2

Mood Swings

"Tell me Doctor, why does my wonderful wife, with her perfect figure and lovely nature, suddenly spit with rage for no obvious reason once a month?"

There are innumerable answers to that question. Most likely she will lay the blame on external events and overlook the upset of chemicals which occurs within her body at the time of menstruation. These chemical changes can produce changes in personality or sudden swings of mood, as menstruation approaches, followed by a return to normality as or after the menstrual flow starts. This is known as the premenstrual syndrome (or, more familiarly, as PMS). Doctors use the word "syndrome" for a group of complaints or symptoms which come together.

The mood swings may vary from a minor nuisance to a major catastrophe. There may be merely an unexpected reaction to a trivial irritation, a hilarious conversation abruptly ended by a cutting or sarcastic remark, a blunt rebuke or just a loss of a sense of humor. On the other end of the scale there may be violent verbal abuse or smashing of things and throwing the nearest object. At the far extreme lies the possibility of suicide, homicide or infanticide. It is easy for an observer to attribute this to a lack of self-control, a mere temperamental outburst or even evidence of the woman's true character. Too rarely are these mood swings properly attributed to the natural ebb and flow of the menstrual hormones over which the woman has such little control.

These premenstrual mood swings are widespread and occur in at least half of all women. But this does mean that there is also another 50% of women who do not experience them at all and do not know what the other half are suffering. Why this fortunate 50% do not suffer is explained in Chapter 14. Men never suffer these changes in hormone levels. The male sex hormones, or chemical messengers, are on an even keel day by day throughout the month, as shown by the levels of follicle stimulating hormone *(FSH)* and testosterone in Figure 2. How different are the levels of the woman's four sex hormones, **follicle stimulating hormone** *(FSH)*, **luteinising hormone** *(LH)*, **estrogen** and **progesterone** which vary day by day throughout the month, as shown in Figure 1. Only a slight imbalance in any of these levels is enough to cause problems for a woman.

"The Premenstrual Syndrome" is used to embrace *any symptoms or complaints which regularly come just before or during early menstruation but are absent at other times of the cycle*. It is the absence of symptoms after menstruation which is so important in this definition. There is an endless list of different symptoms which can be included in this syndrome such as tension, depression, tiredness, irritability, backache, asthma, sinusitis, epilepsy and gain in weight; fortunately no woman suffers from *all* the possible symptoms. All these individual symptoms can also be experienced by men, but in the male they are random occurences, not occuring once every month. It is only in women that we find these symptoms regularly related to menstruation.

Premenstrual syndrome needs to be differentiated from **menstrual distress**. Menstrual distress covers symptoms present during the menstrual cycle with increased intensity before or during menstruation. Such symptoms may be intermittent as with headaches, or continuously present day by day as with anxiety or depression.

Most sufferers of the premenstrual syndrome suffer from more than one symptom at the same time. For instance many sufferers will notice weight-gain and an increase in tension before the onset of a premenstrual headache. The removal of only one symptom, for example by giving a tranquilizer to ease the tension, will be of little help to the gain in weight and the headache.

It is also important to remember that the definition of the premenstrual syndrome requires not only the presence of symptoms related to menstruation, but also the complete absence of these symptoms at other times of the menstrual cycle. It is this absence of symptoms and the change of mood after menstruation back to being a happy, energetic vivacious woman once more, which clinches the diagnosis.

This letter from a patient illustrates the point:

"I have suffered from the usual premenstrual symptoms for five years and my tension, irritability and depression were put down to nerves, but I must say I could never understand this as it was only at certain times of the month that I seem to be so nervous, tense and depressed and lacking confidence. I found that about ten to twelve days before my period I felt as if something was draining out of me and as if something chemical was happening, and so often I tried to pull myself together at this time and it just never worked. I get so irritable and nervous a week before that I just want to shut myself up in a house and I feel as if I can't go out to work and socially I avoid any sort of engagement at this time of the month. At other times I'm O.K."

The exact type and severity of symptoms varies with

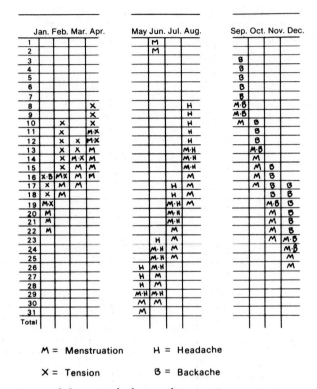

	Jan.	Feb.	Mar.	Apr.
1				
2				
3				
4				
5				
6				
7				
8				X
9				X
10		X		X
11		X		M·X
12		X	X	M·X
13		X	X	M
14		X	M·X	M
15		X	M	M
16	X·B	MX	M	M
17	X	M	M	
18	X	M		
19	M·X			
20	M			
21	M			
22	M			
23				
24				
25				
26				
27				
28				
29				
30				
31				
Total				

	May	Jun.	Jul.	Aug.
1	M			
2	M			
3				
4				
5				
6				
7				
8			H	
9			H	
10			H	
11			H	
12			H	
13			M·H	
14			M·H	
15			M·H	
16			M	
17			H	M
18			H	M
19			M·H	M
20			M·H	
21			M·H	
22			M	
23		H		M
24		M·H		M
25		M·H		M
26	H	M·H		
27	H	M		
28	H	M		
29	M·H	M·H		
30	M	M		
31	M			
Total				

	Sep.	Oct.	Nov.	Dec.
1				
2				
3	B			
4	B			
5	B			
6	B			
7	B			
8	M·B			
9	M·B			
10	M	B		
11		B		
12		B		
13		M·B		
14		M		
15	M	B		
16	M	B		
17	M	B	B	
18		B	B	
19		M·B	B	
20		M	B	
21		M	B	
22		M	B	
23		M	M·B	
24			M·B	
25			M	
26			M	
27				
28				
29				
30				
31				
Total				

M = Menstruation   H = Headache

X = Tension   B = Backache

Figure 3   Menstrual charts diagnostic of premenstrual syndrome

each individual, but in every sufferer her own time-schedule of discomfort is the same, month by month, or rather, cycle by cycle. The easiest tool for recognizing the relationship of symptoms to menstruation and the absence of symptoms at other times of the cycle is the simple chart shown in Figure 3. This is widely used by doctors, and it is easy enough for anyone to copy out for themselves. The letter "M" has been used to represent menstruation, although there are many

	Jan.	Feb.	Mar.	Apr.		May	Jun.	Jul.	Aug.
1	X		X	M					H
2			X	M					
3			X	M		H	H		
4									
5				X					H
6				X		H		H	
7			M			H			
8	X		M·X				H		
9	X		M				H		
10		X	M				H		
11									H
12		M				M		H	
13		M	X	X		M			
14		M				M·H	H		
15		X				M		M	
16	X					M		M	
17	M					M		M	M
18	M					M	M	M	M
19	M	X				M	M	M	M
20		X		X			M	M	M
21			X				M	M	M
22			X			H	M		M
23	X					H	M		
24	X						M·H		
25	X								
26		X							
27				X					
28		X		M		H			H
29				M			H		
30	X			M				H	
31						H			
Total									

M = Menstruation   X = Quarrels

H = Headaches

Figure 4   Menstrual chart with unrelated symptoms

who use the letter "P" for period. (It matters not at all what symbols are used.) Then "X" can be used to denote mood changes or quarrels, "B" for backache and "H" for headache. It is wisest initially to choose the three worst symptoms to chart, and later when these symptoms have been eased consideration can be given to the less serious symptoms. At a glance it will be seen that the quarrels in Figure 4 are not related to menstruation, but occur in a haphazard fashion throughout the month. Such charts are typical of menstrual distress. A full discussion of menstrual patterns and irregularities is contained in Chapter 13.

By using a chart it becomes possible to recognize cyclical mood swings occurring in girls before the onset of menstruation and at the times of missed menstruation during the menopausal years. One mother, a sales executive, who was herself receiving treatment for the premenstrual syndrome, was disturbed to find that her well-behaved daughter of thirteen had occasional "off" days when she would be rude and lazy, which was out of character for her. Then the mother received reports from school that her daughter had occasional rebellious days during which she found it hard to accept discipline but easy to be rude. The mother carefully recorded the dates of her outbursts, which are shown on the chart in Figure 5, with outbursts occurring at intervals of 32–36 days. When later the daughter started to menstruate the timing of her menstrual cycle averaged 35 days. In fact, this mother had diagnosed the premenstrual syndrome before menstruation had started. It is not necessary for ovulation to occur before the premenstrual syndrome develops.

The start of the mood-swings may be quite sudden and the victim may surprise even herself by her own outrageous behavior. It has been described as "a blanket of fog which enfolds me," while a 20-year-old student thought of it as "changing from top gear to bottom in the car." In other cases, the beginning may be quite gradual, symptoms becoming worse day by day. Problems may start at ovulation and last the full fourteen days until menstruation, so that one sufferer felt she had been "crazy for half my life," or it may last for only days or hours before the onset of menstruation. Even if it only lasts for a matter of days it can still be a great source of concern, as one letter-writer described:

	Jan.	Feb.	Mar.	Apr.	May	Jun.
1					X	
2						X
3						X
4						
5						X
6						
7						
8						
9						
10						
11						
12						
13						
14						
15						
16	X					
17	X	X				
18	X	X				
19						
20		X				
21	X	X				
22						
23		X				
24			X			
25			X			
26				X		
27			X	X		
28				X		
29			X	X		
30			X			
31					X	
Total						

13 years old   X = rude or lazy

Figure 5   Chart of adolescent girl with cyclical symptoms before the start of menstruation

"Every month it is the same and the thought of being knocked out for a couple of days each month for the next twenty or so years fills me with a sense of desperation as it is such a waste of days which could be used for living instead of for wallowing in."

Indeed in premenstrual epilepsy the attack may be measured in minutes or hours rather than in days. The symptoms tend to last longer as one approaches the menopause. A 42-year-old teacher wondered if "this gradual lengthening of the negative mood would mean that there may soon be a time when there is no bright spell left at all." It was good to be able to reassure her that, however long the premenstrual mood lasted, there would always be a bright spell once a month after menstruation, for premenstrual symptoms do not start earlier than fourteen days before menstruation, however long or short the menstrual cycle may be.

For many women the onset of menstruation works like a charm, and as the blood flows the relief has been likened to "a cloud lifting" or "the curtain opens again." The very occasional sufferer may even be freed from her symptoms a day or just a few hours before menstruation starts. Yet others may find relief is slower and they may not regain their joy of living until a couple of days after menstruation has finished. When it's over, one may hear a loving husband announce "She's now like the girl I married!"

Medical students are taught that the onset of the premenstrual syndrome is linked with PPPA: puberty, pregnancy, the pill, and after amenorrhoea or absence of menstruation such as occurs after anorexia nervosa or after serious illnesses or accidents. In the young adolescent it may result in an unexpected change of personality. One mother wrote:

"For three weeks of the month our daughter is charming, capable and intelligent, then for the few days before her period she is sharp-tongued, impossible to live with and seems to be boiling with rage."

The premenstrual syndrome may unexpectedly develop when menstruation returns after a pregnancy. If a pregnancy has been complicated by high blood pressure, swelling of the ankles or an abnormally large gain in weight (signs of pre-eclamptic toxemia), or if it has been followed by puerperal or post-natal depression, then the chances are high, ten to one, that the unpleasant premenstrual syndrome will follow in its wake. What is worse, the premenstrual syndrome is likely to increase in severity after each pregnancy, even if the later pregnancies are normal.

The premenstrual syndrome may start when the woman is on the pill, or during the week when she is off it, but complaints are likely to be more marked and the bright and dull days more accentuated when pill-taking ends. Then the woman resumes her normal menstrual cycle, which may well be three or five weeks and not the precise 28 days ordained by the makers of the pill. Marriage is often given as the time at which the premenstrual syndrome started, but in these cases it may be that the observant husband has noticed mood swings and other symptoms and related them to menstruation, when the woman had not noticed the relationship before. Again, pill-taking may have coincided with the marriage.

It is often the outside observer who notices the mood swings first, usually the husband or mother, but occasionally an employer, social worker, friend or daughter. Following a television feature called *Pull Yourself Together, Woman,* a husband wrote:

"I was so startled to recognize in all these cases the symptoms from which my wife has been suffering for the past eight years. The connection with the menstrual cycle may seem less direct but nevertheless the symptoms are heightened in the premenstrual period and free thereafter. Briefly, they include acute anxiety and depression (in any order, as it seems impossible to distinguish cause and effect) manifested by physical symptoms of pressure on the head (variously described as an iron band around the head or a heavy weight at the back of the head) and dizziness; and by psychological symptoms such as agoraphobia, panic, guilt, obsessions and depressions, sometimes to the extent of suicidal notions."

Age and pregnancy are two factors which tend to make the symptoms of the premenstrual syndrome become worse and last longer, so it may be first diagnosed in the thirties. In fact in 1963, Dr. T. Stacy Lloyd, of Virginia, suggested the name "Mid-Thirty Syndrome" for this same collection of symptoms related to menstruation, but this title would be unfair to those who also suffer during adolescence and their twenties.

Recently it has been recognised that premenstrual syndrome often increases in intensity following tubal ligation. Radwanska, Hammond and Berger of Illinois have shown that women have a lower progesterone output from their ovaries after tubal ligation.

This increase in severity is more marked in the years just before the menopause, so much so that all too often the premenstrual mood swings are blamed on to the menopause. A woman of fifty years exclaimed "I've been in the menopause for the last fifteen years, when will it ever end?" It is more likely that she has been suffering from undiagnosed premenstrual syndrome for the last fifteen years.

Fortunately there is an end to this exclusively feminine syndrome, in that when the menopausal changes are complete, menstruation ends and so do the monthly fluctuations of mood and other symptoms. Menopause marks the end of childbearing, ovulation ceases and gradually women's hormones readjust and then progesterone is no longer required. This is the time when one may look forward to an era of serenity.

3

Premenstrual Tension

Tension may be described in many ways, but the tension which occurs in the premenstrual syndrome has three parts to it: depression, tiredness and irritability. These three parts are always present in premenstrual tension although one of them may be more obvious than the others but only temporarily so. Dr. Billig, in 1952, aptly described the depression as "the world looks like a sour apple," the tiredness as a "fall in energy" and the irritability as feeling "crabby," and there are plenty of women who know exactly what he means.

These three symptoms may be interwoven, with each one of equal importance as *Dorothy's* letter shows:

> "Premenstrual tension has been present throughout my reproductive life. I have seen my doctor many times but he has really been unable to help. Perhaps predictably, the condition has grown steadily worse in the years just before the marriage break-up, and much, much worse since. The strain is very great and well-nigh unbearable during the premenstrual time. I do not batter my children physically but I do verbally and I think that that can be almost as damaging, although I do try to explain to them why I behave as I do and apologize for it. The trouble begins as early as twelve to fourteen days after the beginning of the last period; the first sign is a disturbance of sleep. I get violent dreams and often wake

and when it is time to get up feel as though I have· had no rest at all. The other half of the cycle I sleep perfectly soundly. Then I become so tense I positively shake and am so nervous and irritable that I am sorry for anyone who has to live with me. Quite often my heart starts to pound for no obvious reasons, as I have not been running or indulging in any violent exercise. I feel listless and apathetic and often fall asleep during the day, on the other hand the other half of the month I am energetic, hard working and clear headed. The onset of the period releases the tension but triggers off headaches which fluctuate from day to day for a couple of days. I cry at the drop of a hat during all this period and find it hard to deal with any of the many problems objectively. Although I have been very depressed, I have never been put out of action thanks probably to the good professional help. Apart from this misery I am healthy and active and very rarely ill."

Premenstrual tension, popularly abbreviated as "PMT," is only one aspect of the premenstrual syndrome which includes the bodily, or somatic, symptoms as well as the psychological ones.

The tension may come on quite suddenly with an inability to relax and feeling generally uptight. One housewife complained that when she was in this state she seemed to tremble so much that she even had difficulty in threading a needle. Frequently women are shy of mentioning premenstrual tension to their doctor, thinking that it is a common and minor complaint. Instead they seek what is known by the medical profession as a "passport symptom," or a somatic symptom like a headache, backache or 'flu, which they consider is more acceptable to the doctor. One mother wrote:

"When I go to the doctor I am always conscious that I

am not physically ill and so perhaps do not want to tell him all my, to other people, petty feelings. After all one does not want to admit being a failure as a wife and mother."

Sometimes the tension reaches almost manic proportions, with such agitation and restless energy that the woman cannot ease down, she keeps walking up and down, or won't stop talking and just repeats herself endlessly.

One husband was upset because:

"It's no use trying to tell her to relax, she just keeps repeating herself and won't stop talking. New thoughts keep tumbling out. She accuses me of all sorts of things. She just goes on and on and on."

Premenstrual tension, like all other symptoms of the premenstrual syndrome, is always worse at times of stress. None of us can totally free ourselves from the stresses of daily life, such as when extra work is demanded of us because some of those with whom we work are absent or a strike occurs which hampers our normal activities or when friends or neighbors are involved in a car crash or other accident. The usual reaction to any of these stresses will be to cause an increase in the premenstrual tension when the time of the next menstruation approaches. On the other hand good news will tend to ease the tension, and a winning bet or lottery ticket can be most beneficial in relieving premenstrual tension, but only for a month or two.

DEPRESSION

The depression may be so mild that the actual word is not used or is even denied. However, the woman may admit to feeling fed up, down in the dumps, that she can't laugh easily and has difficulty in smiling, or that the whole world is against her but nobody cares. On the other hand premenstrual depression may range to the other extreme with the ever-present possibility of suicide, and this is a risk which should be fully appreciated.

One husband wrote describing his wife's depression:

"I feel her life is at risk; she dreads these times so much it colors her whole life. She feels there is no hope."

A mother described her 20-year-old daughter's depression:

"These occurrences are so regular that for years I have associated them with periods. But when she approaches her doctor, usually in a state of panic, she is either told to go away and pull herself together, or is given tranquilizers and on at least three occasions she has taken the lot and has had to have her stomach pumped out. When she is in this state she often proves violent and smashes things or hits her boyfriend. She also swallows vast quantities of alcohol and then sometimes cuts her wrists, always in the wrong direction. When she is herself after a period she is such a nice, kind and good-natured person."

A Washington, D.C. secretary ended her full description of premenstrual depression with the statement:

"The sad thing is that although suicidal thoughts cross my mind at this time, I am a very happy person ordinarily."

The MacKinnons, a husband and wife team of doctors, showed as long ago as 1956 that successful suicides predominated during the premenstruum. Studies into attempted suicides in hospitals in London and Delhi and among the Samaritans in Los Angeles have all confirmed that half of all women's attempts at suicide are made during the four days immediately before or the first four days of menstruation.

Although women make more attempts at suicide than men, the men succeed more frequently, but this masculine success rate gradually disappears after the age of 50 years. Dr. John Pollitt, speaking at the Royal Society of Medicine in 1976, suggested that

> "perhaps one reason for the female's lack of success is that the majority of attempts are made during the premenstrual phase or menstruation. Killing oneself is not easy; success requires careful planning. Women in the premenstrual phase show a marked tendency to be careless, thoughtless, unpunctual, forgetful and absent-minded. This inefficiency at a time when they are more likely to try to end their lives may result in a disproportionate failure."

Every suicidal gesture should be taken seriously, as just before and during menstruation a sufferer's mood may deteriorate so suddenly that an attempt may be made at a most unexpected moment. The attempt may end the life, even though it was only intended as a cry for help, or it may result in permanent damage even harder to cope with than the condition at the time of the attempt. Drug overdoses may result in permanent liver or kidney damage, and when a woman throws herself under a train or from a high window the scarred face and broken limbs are ever-present reminders of the event which made life so intolerable. One patient produced her diaries with a record of 40 overdose attempts, each one had needed hospital admission and had occurred during her premenstruum, those four fateful days before menstruation.

Edith, a 24-year-old personal assistant, wrote:

"On December 6th, realizing how dangerous the pre-menstrual effects were, I felt in great need of help. Un-fortunately my group meeting was during this time and did not help me at all. After the meeting I rushed home, hid from my boyfriend whom I saw downtown, and intended again to overdose. Fortunately two friends arrived on the scene and by the time they left it was all over and I had started to menstruate."

Depression can be an emotion, such as when we hear of the death of a near friend or other bad news, but it can also be an illness when it affects all the bodily functions as well. The symptoms of a depressive illness are just the same as in premenstrual depression, the only difference being in the timing. Whereas in a depressive illness the symptoms are present throughout the month, although possibly more severe as menstruation approaches, in premenstrual depres-sion the woman is her normal happy, energetic self after menstruation. Premenstrual depression increases with age after 26 years and is common among single women.

Depression is best thought of as a disease of "loss," for there is a loss of happiness, interests and enthusiasm, loss of memory, energy, sleep and sexual arousal. One feels a loss of security and adequacy and a loss of the powers of concen-tration, so that it becomes difficult to read a book or watch a television play. There is a loss of self-control, and an in-ability to make decisions or to control one's tears, behavior and appetite. There is a loss of insight and an inability to realize, in the case of premenstrual depression, that very shortly the symptoms will pass during the course of menstru-ation and that there will be a return to normality.

TIREDNESS

"What worries me most is that I get so slow and stupid before my periods." This comment by a journalist is echoed by many who find the lethargy, exhaustion and prostration so difficult to cope with during the premenstruum. The "can't-be-bothered" attitude takes over and disrupts the program for the day until in the end "everything goes."

Frances, a 32-year-old working mother, hated the tiredness most and wrote:

"The worst and most worrying symptom is the feeling of apathy which descends on me; all physical and mental activity becomes a real effort and all I want to do is curl up in a corner away from everyone and all my responsibilities. I find it quite frightening that I cannot think clearly or quickly and feel mentally dulled. These symptoms get increasingly worse and a couple of days before a period I feel quite ill. The first day of a period I feel a bit headachy and tired, but then it is like a weight being lifted off me and for two weeks or so I feel really fine."

Again the tiredness may vary in severity from the typist who fills her wastebasket with her typing errors to the executive who feels unable to compose letters and stares all day at a blank sheet of paper. A mother of two boys, aged one and three years old wrote:

"When I am bad I stay in bed all day. One day last holiday I felt so bad I could not bear to lift my sons or get them dressed so the poor children had to stay in bed the whole day. I just cried and told them how sorry I was that I could not help them at all. I fear the little ones who have known me like this may grow up into disturbed children, but I promise you I'm quite normal at other times in my cycle."

One woman, as yet unknown to me, asked for an appointment, and when describing her tiredness added:

"I seem to be in a daze on those days, can't do anything right – more than once I've crossed the road to go to the bathroom and have found myself in the Gents."

Another housewife confessed that:

"Just before a period, for about ten days a sleepiness takes me over and all I want to do is sit down and sleep, so therefore no housework or proper cooking gets done."

It is the premenstrual tiredness which is responsible for the drop in mental ability before menstruation. At one boarding school it was possible to study 1,561 weekly grades of schoolchildren and compare them with the previous week's grades. Each grade covered the total scores of some seven to twelve different subjects. During the premenstrual week there was an average drop of 10% compared with a compensatory rise of 20% during the week immediately following menstruation, as shown in Figure 6. This effect is also evident in high school and college level examination results.

IRRITABILITY

It is those who are nearest to a sufferer of premenstrual irritability that suffer most, and this is usually not only the nearest but also the dearest, which means the husband, children or parents. As one wife said:

"Pity those around me when the least things upset me, I hate everyone, shouting and picking quarrels, and the whole world gets on my nerves and I can only look at it with a jaundiced eye."

Premenstrual irritability is commoner in the married woman, and the husband naturally has problems trying to

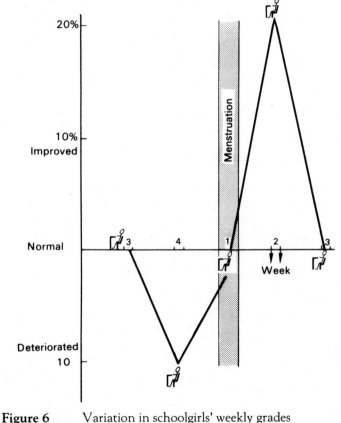

Figure 6   Variation in schoolgirls' weekly grades with menstruation

calm a supersensitive, edgy, irrational and agitated woman during these days of each cycle. Too many end up with visits to the marriage guidance counselor or in divorce.

The following three quotations taken from letters received suggest that the husband has obviously suffered as much as his wife:

"I have been suffering from premenstrual tension for some years now, and recently it came to its height. In July I was in my usual depressed state and, being angry, I didn't know what to do with myself; I just lost my temper and for the thousandth time I kicked the door and required forty stitches in my leg. My husband is at his wits' end not knowing what to do with me, not knowing what I'm going to do next and is ready to leave me after being married only eighteen months. I keep telling him that I'll be good the next time, but I never am and just can't control myself."

"Last Saturday I deliberately smashed all the dishes after clearing the table. I started menstruating in the evening. My general practitioner puts it down to my Irish temper. I get so depressed, hateful, horrid, tired, stay in bed, shout and I could go on and on like this. It is my husband who asked me to write for help."

"At thirty-two there is very little hope for me except the change; I have a history of suicide attempts, child and husband bashing and many fights with a long-suffering doctor, who has been accused by me of many crimes, neglect and attempted manslaughter amongst them; at my worst I have taken many prescribed anti-depressants in massive overdoses."

If one sees a patient shortly after an aggressive outburst, like those described in the last three letters, it is possible to get full details of the time at which food has been taken during the day. It is a common finding that the irritability is always worse when, in addition to the closeness of menstruation, there has been a long interval since the last meal, causing the blood sugar level to fall (see discussion on blood sugar levels, page 131). When patients are asked at what time of day their irritability rockets, it is usually in the late morning if breakfast has been missed, or when preparing the evening meal or waiting for the husband's return if he is later than usual. Often the wife has only had a sandwich, or possibly just cheese and an apple at midday, and is then at her wits' end, having eaten nothing else in anticipation of an evening meal with her husband. These sudden explosive outbursts of irritability or aggression can usually be helped by ensuring that regular small meals are taken at intervals of three hours. In two recent cases of murder and one of infanticide it was noted that no food had been taken for nine hours.

At the height of the tension there may be true confusion so that the woman is unaware of her actions or surroundings. Indeed she may bitterly refute any action, for she has no memory of it. The following notes made by a patient show how extreme the confusion may be and how it may well represent temporary insanity.

"From the 4th onwards severe depression with secretive confusion. On the 7th I planned to kill my mother and myself. I wrote suicide notes to all concerned and took certain prescribed drugs that I thought would work. I do not know whether I would have done it as my friend, with whom I have a good relationship, discovered that they were missing and flushed them down the toilet. It took quite a few days before I realized how bizarre the whole episode was. The loss of appetite, need for alcohol, aggression, lack of interest and swollen glands continued until menstruation started on the 9th. These notes are written on the 18th, when my mind is clear."

It is not surprising that premenstrual tension with its irritability and confusion frequently leads to brushes with the law. There are those cases of assault where in a sudden fit of temper the woman throws a rolling-pin at her neighbor, a typewriter at her boss or tries to bite off a policeman's ear. There are the cases of baby-battering, husband-hitting and homicide as seen in the cases already quoted. Becoming drunk and disorderly when under the influence of alcohol or drugs may also lead to charges of assault. In France it is recognized that premenstrual tension may be so acute and so violent as to be classed as "temporary insanity" in courts of law.

In Britain a survey of 156 newly committed women prisoners revealed that half had committed their crime during the paramenstruum, and in fact the premenstrual syndrome was present in two thirds of these women who committed their crime during the paramenstruum. Theft accounted for the highest proportion, with 56% of crimes being committed during the paramenstruum, while the alcoholics charged with being "drunk and disorderly" were a close second.

The Parisian police noticed early this century that 84% of crimes of violence by women had been committed during the premenstruum or menstruation. This was confirmed by a similar study in New York which showed that 62% of crimes of violence occurred during the premenstruum.

Dr. Morton and his colleagues working in Westfield State Prison, Bedford Hills, New York, showed that it was worthwhile treating the inmates of prisons and reformatories if they suffered from the premenstrual syndrome. He found that treatment resulted in an increased work output, less punishment for disobeying rules and an increase in general morale.

The question may well be asked here: what benefit will a woman gain from a prison sentence or fine if she is unable to control her premenstrual irritability or confusion?

4

Waterlogged

For some women, the days from ovulation to menstruation are characterized by a gain in weight, with a feeling of bloatedness and heaviness. This is due to an accumulation of water in the tissues and cells of the body, because only part of all the water that is taken in during those two weeks is passed out from the body, some remains and gradually accumulates. Not only is water retained but so is sodium, while potassium is lost. It should be stressed that water-retention is only one of the many symptoms of the premenstrual syndrome, and many women never experience it at all even though they may suffer from severe premenstrual tension or other symptoms.

The commonest sign of water being retained in the body is an increase of weight, which may average 4 to 7 lbs above the normal weight (Figure 7), but of course it may well be more, even 10 to 12 lbs. The normal weight is that which is taken during the postmenstruum and gains and losses of up to 3 lbs are usually considered within normal limits for women. Dr. William Thomas MD, of Chicago, has documented a case of one woman who gained between 12 and 14 lbs each premenstruum and then lost it altogether with an excessive output of 9 pints of urine on the first day of menstruation, the excessive urine output continuing for the next few days of menstruation. Those who regularly gain and lose very large amounts of water periodically are sometimes diagnosed as suffering from "cyclical idiopathic edema."

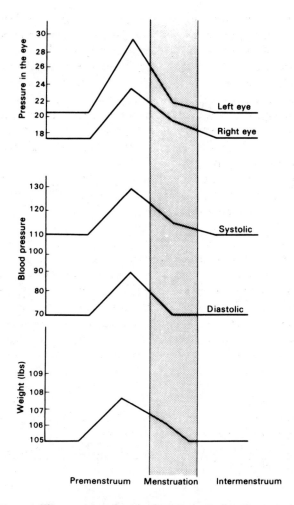

Figure 7   Fluctuations during the menstrual cycle
in weight, blood pressure and pressure
in the eye of a sufferer of the
premenstrual syndrome

The early workers on the premenstrual syndrome believed that the premenstrual weight gain was an index of the severity of the premenstrual symptoms, but this is definitely not the case. Dr. Bruce and Professor Russell examined thirty-four women at Maudsley Hospital, London, who complained of premenstrual symptoms, carefully measuring their weights and the amount of fluids they took in and the amount they passed out, and found no relationship. In fact they wrongly concluded that the premenstrual syndrome was a purely psychological condition.

Apart from the gain in weight, the water retention shows itself in the different tissues, with varying effects, as experienced by *Gladys* who wrote:

"The pattern of 5 lbs weight rise at period times makes me so bloated that it turns me out of my favorite slacks and makes me feel ready to burst. My breasts become enlarged and sore needing a larger size bra, my eyes sink back and I get dark rings under the eyes. There is extreme fatigue, both physical, so that I can hardly put one foot before the other, and mental, so that I feel incapable of dealing with the children I teach. I am subject to quite black depressions caused by trivial things going wrong. I get throbbing and severe headaches in the week preceding the period and always during the first three days of bleeding. I do a full-time job, look after the home and three children, go to evening classes, I also paint and do flower arranging, so you see I do try to fight it."

BREAST SORENESS

Complaints of breast soreness with enlargement and tender nipples are common, and all too frequently this leads to fear that this may be a sign of cancer of the breast. It is definitely not related to cancer in any way. It is more that the breast tissue is getting ready in the hope that following ovulation a pregnancy will occur and the breasts will be needed for breast feeding, rather than as mere sex symbols.

FLUID RETENTION

The extra water in the tissues can cause the ankles and the fingers to swell so that shoes have to be discarded and the wedding-ring removed. There may be swelling of the gums so that dentures no longer fit. The skin coarsens and becomes blotchy, contact lenses won't fit and the hair becomes lank. One model, who refused to accept work during the premenstruum, said:

> "I look my very worst, my skin won't take make-up, my face goes stiff and I can't move gracefully with those extra pounds of weight!"

The exact place where the water accumulates varies in different women and at different times in their life. The most severe symptoms result from water accumulating in a small unstretchable area, such as when water accumulates in the labyrinth of the inner ear and causes dizziness, when it enters the eyeball causing a raised pressure inside the eye and severe pain, and when it occurs inside the unyielding bony skull causing headaches. The sinuses are air spaces within the bones of the face where air enters through a small entrance which is lined with cells of the mucus membrane; when these are engorged and swollen the entrance to the sinus is blocked causing stale air to accumulate in the sinus resulting in sinus headaches or "vacuum headaches." Water can also accumulate in the discs between the vertebrae of the spine, causing backache.

Sometimes there is a widespread distribution of the

extra water which produces vague symptoms in the muscles, joints and soft tissues, causing generalized rheumatic pains, abdominal bloating and heaviness. The water is always in the cells or in the fluid between the cells. It is never free, although one patient imagined she could hear the water "splashing within her abdomen." When the extra water accumulates in the fat and subcutaneous tissues there can be an appreciable gain in weight without any other complaints. This is most likely to happen in obese women.

LOCATING THE WATER

The actual site where the cells become swollen may vary from time to time depending on such factors as (1) anatomical abnormality (2) heredity (3) injury and (4) infection. Thus a premenstrual sinus headache is more likely to occur in a woman whose cartilage in her nose is bent. Water is readily attracted to cells which have recently been injured or infected, so that after a fracture of the leg or arm it is usual to notice premenstrual swelling there for some months afterwards. If someone has recently had pneumonia it is likely that, if water retention occurs during the premenstruum, this may cause a return of the cough or breathlessness.

This water retention, is often blamed for the depression and other symptoms which accompany it. *Helen*, a 27-year-old unmarried accountant, wrote:

"I start to get tender, swollen breasts, usually 14 days (ovulation?) before the beginning of menstruation and I gain several pounds in weight. This makes me depressed and bad-tempered and when you feel like that you can't help getting annoyed with everyone around you."

Many of the symptoms of water retention are characteristically worse in the early morning, often waking the patient from her sleep. This is especially so with migraine and with the acute pain in the eyeball, mimicking glaucoma; and asthma where there is swelling of the lining cells of the small tubes of the lung. Some people are awakened by a feeling of pins and needles, and perhaps numbness of their fingers. This is because the nerve passes from the arm through a narrow bony tunnel at the wrist, and when the surrounding cells are swollen and waterlogged this nerve becomes constricted. It is this which causes the odd sensations in the fingers, and it may be called "carpal tunnel syndrome."

Nowadays, when we have many drugs which help to increase the amount of urine passed, these would seem to be a simple answer to the problem of water retention. Unfortunately the problem is not quite so simple. Although these drugs or diuretics can get rid of water, extra water forms again quickly; it is rather like baling water from a boat with a hole in it. It is better to bung up the hole and prevent further water entering than merely to keep baling. Just as the balers get tired, so do the water tablets. So the temptation then is to use stronger and even stronger drugs to get rid of more and more water. But as mentioned at the beginning of the chapter, the problem is not only that water accumulates but also that potassium is lost. Diuretics cause water and more potassium to pass away in the urine so unless sufficient potassium is added one may cause a marked lowering of the blood potassium level resulting in an increase in the tiredness and possibly also weakness of the legs. Doctors can do an estimation of blood potassium level to know how much potassium is circulating in the blood at a given moment, but this does not tell you how much potassium is present in the cells or in the fluid between the cells, which is really what matters.

Another problem is that water retention does not cause premenstrual tension, depression, tiredness or irritability, so none of these symptoms will be relieved by diuretics. Actually diuretics are useful only in the short term until progesterone treatment can be given, or in the mild case where it is used sparingly with the addition of extra potassium.

One often meets patients who have received diuretics continuously for many years and have become dehydrated. If diuretics are then stopped suddenly the patients complain bitterly of feeling bloated within a day or two of stopping. These patients need to be persuaded to gradually tail off their diuretics by using them every other day, starting immediately after menstruation. After a month or two it may be possible to decrease the dose to every third or fourth day until it is only used when the weight gain is really marked.

When a woman starts to gain weight there is the very natural temptation to start dieting. If her weight is above the ideal weight for her age and height this is all to the good, but she needs to be careful which diet she chooses. Not for her a diet of fruit juice and liquids only, as this will merely increase the water retention. If she tries to solve the problem by missing out meals, she risks the possibility that her blood sugar level will drop abnormally low, thus increasing the depression and irritability. Dr. Jerome W. Conn of Michigan was the first to describe in 1955 a condition of primary aldosteronism, known as Conn's syndrome. He probably knows more than anyone about water, salt and potassium balance, and he has suggested that the body's reaction to a low blood sugar level is related to the amount of potassium in the cells. He has shown that the blood sugar level can be improved by correcting the potassium deficiency which may be present.

On the other hand if a woman is already below or at the average weight for her height and age, it is important for her to appreciate that the gain in weight is due to excess water and try to limit her fluids to four cups daily and restrict salt, rather than to try counting calories and restricting food.

5

Monthly Headaches

Many women like to jump on the bandwagon and claim that their own particular variety of headache only comes at period time. Undoubtedly menstruation is the most frequent time for migraine attacks in women, as shown in Figure 8 in which the times of 935 migraine attacks are shown in relation to the days of the menstrual cycle. On the other hand those who can produce a three-month record showing a regular and definite relationship of the headache to menstruation have a much better chance of obtaining relief from progesterone treatment. In Figure 9 it will be seen that Isobel's headaches last between 7 and 10 days before each period and are preceded by symptoms of tension, which ease off during the menstruation. Joan gives a different picture: her headaches only last one or two days, and there is no premenstrual tension, but the headaches all tend to come around the time of menstruation. Kathleen seems to have headaches every ten or twelve days, occasionally they do coincide with menstruation, but often they just come at any time. It is unlikely that Kathleen will benefit from hormonal treatment.

Characteristically, monthly headaches which are likely to benefit from treatment with specific hormones such as progesterone are those showing a definite relationship to menstruation in a three-month record, and those headaches which started either at puberty, after a pregnancy or while on the pill. These women are likely to be free from headaches after the fourth month of pregnancy, and may well look back to the later months of pregnancy as the only time in their life when they knew what it was like to be free from headaches. But alas, these same women are also likely to say

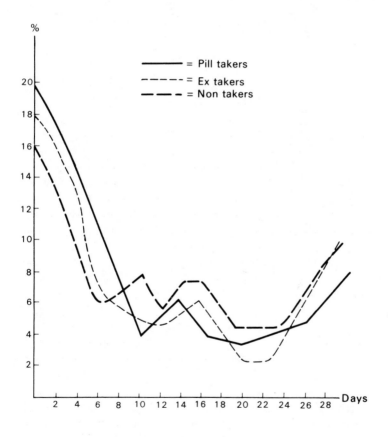

Figure 8 935 migraine attacks in relation to the menstrual cycle

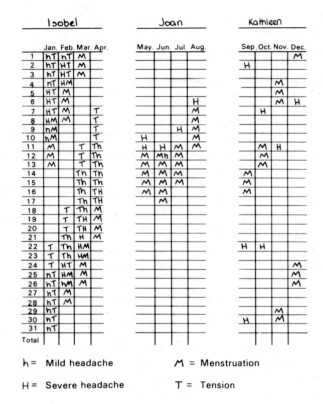

	Isobel				Joan				Kathleen			
	Jan.	Feb.	Mar.	Apr.	May.	Jun.	Jul.	Aug.	Sep.	Oct.	Nov.	Dec.
1	hT	hT	M									M
2	hT	HT	M						H			
3	hT	HT	M									
4	nT	HM									M	
5	HT	M									M	
6	HT	M						H			M	H
7	HT	M		T				M		H		
8	HM	M		T				M				
9	nM			T			H	M				
10	hM			T	H			M				
11	M		T	Th	H	H	M	M		M	H	
12	M		T	Th	M	Mh	M			M		
13	M		T	Th	M	M	M			M		
14			Th	Th	M	M	M		M			
15			Th	Th	M	M	M		M			
16			Th	TH	M	M			M			
17			Th	TH	M							
18		T	Th	M								
19		T	TH	M								
20		T	TH	M								
21		Th	H	M								
22	T	Th	HM						H	H		
23	T	Th	HM									
24	T	HT	M									M
25	nT	HM	M									M
26	hT	hM	M									M
27	hT	M										
28	hT	M										
29	hT										M	
30	nT								H		M	
31	nT											
Total												

h = Mild headache   M = Menstruation

H = Severe headache   T = Tension

Figure 9   Headaches in relation to menstruation

that immediately after the pregnancy the headaches returned worse than ever.

Women who find their headaches become worse while on the pill, or who have a tendency to headaches on the first or second day after stopping the course of pills, are likely to have menstrual headaches responsive to treatment. The majority of these women with menstrually related headaches are also likely to find that after the menopause most of their problems come to an end.

The three common types of headaches related to menstruation are (1) sinus or vacuum headaches (2) tension headaches and (3) migraine.

VACUUM HEADACHES

It is better to speak of "vacuum headaches" rather than "sinus headaches" as the latter are likely to be confused with the headache resulting from true sinusitis, which is due to infected material getting lodged in the sinuses. On the other hand the vacuum headaches are due to swelling of the cells at the entrance to the sinus, blocking the entry so that the stale air accumulates inside. These women may know that a headache is on the way when their nasal passages become blocked and it is difficult to breathe through one of their nostrils. There is tenderness or pressure over the sinuses, which are situated in the cheek bone and over the eyes. (Figure 10) The pain that results is made worse by bending down, and may last from one to seven days. In addition there may well be other signs of waterlogging such as a gain in weight, bloated abdomen, shortness of breath or swollen ankles or fingers. These women would be wise to restrict their fluid intake to four cups of liquid daily and may benefit from nasal decongestants.

TENSION HEADACHES

The tension headaches usually have a slow onset, so that the woman who is trying to chart it for the record may be uncertain whether the pain in the head is bad enough to call a headache. It usually starts after the beginning of the symptoms of premenstrual tension, irritability, tiredness or depression and eases off gradually during the course of menstruation. The pain from tension headaches has been described as "like a steel band enclosing my head" or "like a heavy weight on top of my head." (Figure 10) These women will find that the usual analgesics, such as aspirin or paracetamol, will only give ease for about four hours and then the headache returns again, and the analgesic must be repeated. Treatment with progesterone (see Chapter 18) is most valuable for this type of headache, and it also relieves the other symptoms of the premenstrual syndrome.

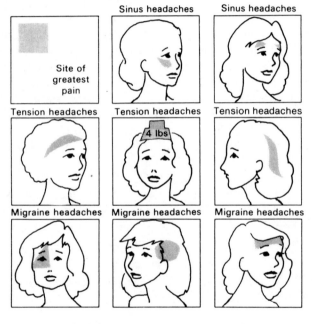

Figure 10   Sites of greatest pain in menstrual headaches

MIGRAINE

Doctors like to divide migraine into two varieties, the classical and the common type. In the classical variety the patient has a warning or 'aura' lasting about 20 minutes before the onset of a severe headache. This aura may be of sudden flashes of lights, brightly colored stars or stripes, a patch of blindness, or there may be sensations of pins and needles in the tongue, side of face or hands and legs. Many people suffer both classical and common migraine at different times over the years. Common migraine has no aura and begins gradually, increasing in severity. The migraine may be accompanied by nausea or vomiting and extreme prostration and is likely to last between 24 and 48 hours, although some unlucky women find it lasts even longer.

Most migraine sufferers have a family history with a parent, brothers, sisters and uncles or aunts also suffering, so they do start life with a predisposition to migraine. Nevertheless there are those among them whose attacks are related to menstruation and can benefit from simple advice and possibly also progesterone treatment.

In order to help women who have frequent or severe migraine attacks it is helpful to have full details of all they have been doing, and the times at which all foods have been consumed. In practice an attack form, like that shown in Figure 11, proves valuable and helps to isolate an individual trigger factor. The trigger factor is the last straw which decides exactly when a migraine is going to occur in a susceptible woman. It is often the result of either going too long without food, so that there is a drop in the blood sugar level, or eating certain foods to which the sufferer is sensitive.

TOO LONG WITHOUT FOOD

When women are asked what sort of things start a migraine attack they often mention travel, theater going, and the day after a great event, such as when they have been working hard for several days preparing for a rummage sale, a wedding or special party. If the attack forms have been carefully filled in it is usually easy to spot if the migraine has been

Name................................	Date.................................
	Day of week.........................
	Time of onset ....
	Duration ....
Day of cycle........................	Days before next menstruation......

During the 24 hours *before* an attack:—

(1) Did you have any special worry, overwork or shock?
(2) What had you done during the day?
     Normal work?
     Unusual activity?
     Extra tired?
(3) What food had you eaten and when?

Breakfast.......................	Time................................
....	
Mid-morning....................	Time................................
....	
Lunch	Time................................
....	
Mid-afternoon...................	Time................................
....	
Supper	Time................................
....	
Evening	Time................................
....	
Bedtime	Time................................
....	

Figure 11   An attack form useful for isolating
trigger factors in migraine

caused by too long an interval without food. Generally speaking five hours between meals is long enough for most women leading a normal energetic life, but women with premenstrual syndrome will find that over three hours is too long an interval without food. An overnight interval exceeding thirteen hours is usually considered the limit. After this length of time susceptible women, probably those already born with the tendency to migraine, will find they develop a headache. This explains why travel often causes a headache, for with frequent delays and long distances travelled, eating is often left for longer than usual. Similarly if one is busy with preparations for special events the food may all too easily be forgotten. And if you are giving the party, how easy it is to ensure that your guests have plenty to eat but forget to take any food yourself.

Furthermore, one must consider not only the interval between meals but the amount of energy expended during the interval, as the more energy is exerted, the quicker the blood sugar level falls. Overnight fasting is often the cause of a migraine attack on waking, and there are those migraine sufferers who say they cannot sleep long on holidays or at the weekend because they only wake up with a headache. Migraine is likely to occur when the evening meal is followed by some energetic sport or a brisk walk and no further food is taken before retiring to bed.

An example of this was noted in a receptionist, who was also a keen skater, and normally had her evening meal at 6:30 P.M. On Thursdays she would be off to the rink for three hours of energetic enjoyment before retiring, but had no food after the evening meal. Every four to five weeks she would wake with a migraine on Friday mornings. The attacks occurred during the paramenstruum, but were triggered off by the long interval without food and the energetic skating.

Full information about the effect of a drop in blood sugar level is given on pages 131–134. If the attack forms suggest that the woman has had too long an interval without food, or has been too energetic for the amount of food she has had, it would suggest that the sudden drop in blood sugar may have triggered the attack. The question of treatment then becomes obvious: avoid fasting, remember to have an extra cookie with the morning and afternoon coffee or tea. Remember, too, that proteins, such as meat, fish and eggs, will keep the blood sugar up longer, while glucose sweets only cause a short, sharp rise in blood sugar level followed by a quick drop, and thus provide only a temporary benefit.

FOODS CAUSING MIGRAINE

Other women whose migraine attacks are not because of fasting may find that they are sensitive to certain foods, the commonest of which are cheese, chocolate, alcohol and citrus fruits, but a few are sensitive to ripe bananas, pork, onions, fish and gluten. In these cases the migraine attacks do not occur immediately after the specific food has been eaten, but some 12 to 36 hours later. This is because the attack occurs, not when the food is digested in the stomach, but rather when it is later broken down in the liver. In the liver these end products are finally broken down by the action of special chemicals known as 'enzymes' and it would seem that if one particular enzyme is not present then a wrong chemical action occurs, releasing substances capable of opening wide the blood vessels of the brain. These substances are known as 'vaso-dilating amines'; two common ones are tyramine, which is present in cheese, and phenylethylamine, which is present in alcohol and chocolate, but there are also many other vaso-dilating amines, which can form from the wrong breakdown of everyday foods.

During the paramenstruum it seems that some women's sensitivity to vaso-dilating amines may be increased so that although they are able to take small amounts of, say, cheese, after menstruation, as menstruation approaches or during menstruation even a minute amount is sufficient to provoke an attack.

Women who come into this category would be wise if they try to avoid the foods to which they are sensitive, remembering always that it is an individual problem. Foods which cause attacks in one individual will not necessarily cause attacks in another migraine sufferer. However, as mentioned earlier, there are often other members of the family who also suffer from migraine, so it is well worthwhile having a "gathering of the clan" at which all blood relations who suffer from migraine can swop their ideas on the foods which they feel are detrimental to them. Often a common food can be discovered to which all members are sensitive.

Those who are sensitive to cheese will be happy to learn that tyramine is not present in cream or cottage cheese, but only develops on maturing, so among the particular cheeses to be avoided are Stilton, Cheddar, Parmesan and processed cheeses. However they should be aware that mature cheese is often hidden in quiches, mornay sauce and Italian dishes.

Red wine, sherry, port and champagne are probably the worst alcohols for causing migraine, but it is often possible to take a single glass of white wine with food without any after-effects. It is also worth considering the difference between grape and grain alcohols, for more people are sensitive to grape alcohols than to the grain alcohols like beer and whiskey.

Chocolate is often added to rich fruit cakes or ginger cakes to give a good color, and to coffee dishes to increase the flavor, so those who are sensitive to chocolate should be on their guard. Plain dark chocolate is more likely to provoke an attack than milk chocolate. And how easy it is for those sensitive to citrus fruits to forget that this also includes mandarins and tangerines.

6

Recurrent Problems

My interest in the premenstrual syndrome was first aroused within a few days of qualifying as a doctor, and whilst working as a fill-in for a general practitioner. In the early hours of the morning a call was received from a 34-year-old mother of three children, who had an acute attack of asthma. The husband, who opened the door, was most apologetic for calling the doctor out at such an hour, but added "Unfortunately it happens every month except when she's pregnant." The woman certainly had a severe asthmatic attack and was quickly given an injection to ease her breathing. Driving home, the husband's words recalled my own migraine which also occurred once a month, just before menstruation, and the only time of freedom had been during my pregnancies. Later that day, a visit to the patient revealed that her first attack of asthma had occurred at the age of 17 years, coinciding with her first period, and she had an attack of asthma with each menstruation. The medical textbooks did not mention this possibility, but Dr. Raymond Greene, who had helped me with my migraine, suggested that this patient should also be treated with progesterone. In those days the doctor gave the injections, and during that first month while giving the asthma patient her daily injections, I came across another woman with premenstrual asthma, two with premenstrual epilepsy and one with premenstrual migraine. So did the story of the premenstrual syndrome begin. In those days the emphasis was essentially on bodily ailments, with less appreciation of the tension and other psychological symptoms.

The only way to identify a chronic recurring symptom as being part of the premenstrual syndrome is to chart it carefully together with the dates of menstruation for at least three months. If this was done more frequently there would be many more women whose asthma, epilepsy, migraine and a host of other complaints would be identified as menstrually related and would then be eligible for relief by progesterone therapy. At present the list of symptoms which can, in some individuals, be related to menstruation proves to be endless and certainly covers all the systems of the body, so that all specialists, no matter what their discipline, are likely to come across its effects. In fact many of the symptoms are among the commonest that the specialist is called upon to treat. For instance the neurologist sees most patients with headaches and epilepsy, the dermatologist sees many patients with acne, boils and herpes, and so on.

Women with bodily, or somatic, symptoms related to menstruation will have the usual characteristics of the premenstrual syndrome, they will have the onset at puberty, after pregnancy or use of the pill, or when menstruation resumes after a few months absence. They will be free from symptoms in later pregnancy, and symptoms will be eased after the menopause. There will be a high number whose symptoms start after a pregnancy complicated by pre-eclamptic toxemia or following postnatal depression.

Whilst it will never be possible to give a list of all the possible symptoms which on occasion may be included in the premenstrual syndrome, the common ones can be discussed. (Figure 12)

The premenstrual *asthma* appears to be caused by water retention in the cells lining the smaller tubes of the lung which become swollen and prevent the free entry of air into the minute air sacs. Thus the cause is not necessarily allergic, in fact these patients do not all respond to sodium cromoglycate (Intal) inhalers as do those whose asthma has a definite allergic basis. Premenstrual asthma is particularly common in women in their thirties and forties. Usually the women will volunteer that their attacks are brought on by

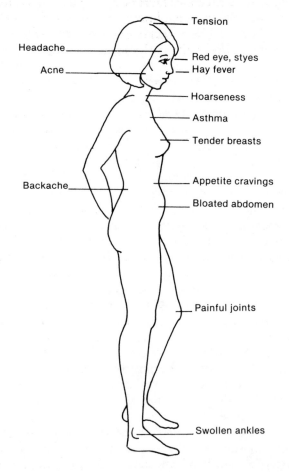

Figure 12   Common symptoms of the premenstrual syndrome

stress and tension, but they may not yet have related it to premenstrual tension. In the special asthma clinics in hospitals it is usual to find that about one third of women of childbearing years have menstrually related asthma. Two women, aged eighteen and forty-two, have been treated at the Premenstrual Syndrome Clinic, University College Hospital, London. They had both had over twenty admissions to intensive care units for acute asthma, until an alert ward sister noticed that the attacks always occurred premenstrually. Both have since been free from asthma on progesterone treatment.

One of the most satisfying experiences is to be able to diagnose and treat a woman with premenstrual *epilepsy*. They can be treated with progesterone and freed from all anti-convulsant tablets with their many and unpleasant side effects. Furthermore, in Britain if they are not taking anti-convulsant drugs and have been three years without an epileptic fit, they have the joy of having their driving licenses returned to them. It seems that premenstrual epilepsy is often a culminating symptom on top of gradually increasing tension and headache, so these patients do have a warning that an attack is imminent. There may also be marked weight gain, but this is not always so. Often the final precipitating trigger, immediately prior to an attack, is a long interval without food.

Laura, 28 years, with one child, set off on holiday having had only a light breakfast at 8:00 A.M. Her husband drove some 300 miles stopping only to ask the way. When she arrived at her hotel she had a nasty headache and while she was unpacking at about 5:00 P.M. she had an epileptic fit. She started menstruating the next day. She later agreed that there had been mounting tension during the previous week which she had attributed to trying to finish all the necessary jobs in time for her holiday.

Name __Margaret__

	Jan.	Feb.	Mar.	Apr.	May	Jun.
1		M				
2						
3	X					
4						
5	M					M
6	M					M
7	M				M	M
8	M				M	M
9	M				M	M
10						M
11						M
12						M
13						
14						
15					M	
16					M	
17					M	
18					MX	
19				M	M	
20				M	M	
21		X		M	M	
22				M		
23			M	M		
24			M	M		
25			M			
26			M			
27			M			
28	M				*	
29	M					
30	MX					
31	M					
Total						

Name __Nancy__

	Jan.	Feb.	Mar.	Apr.	May	Jun.	Jul.
1							
2							
3			X				
4				X			
5				M			
6			MX	M			
7			M	MX			
8			M	M			
9		X	MX	M			
10							
11		X					
12		M					
13	M	MX					
14	M	M					M
15	M	M					M
16	M	M				M	M
17	M	M				M	M
18	M	MX				M	
19	M	M				M	
20	M					M	
21						M	
22							
23							
24							
25							
26							
27							
28							
29					*		
30							
31							
Total							

Margaret is 27 yrs old with 2 children, onset after 1st pregnancy

Nancy is 28 yrs old, onset at puberty

M = menstruation
X = epileptic attack
* = progesterone treatment started

Figure 13　　Charts of two patients with premenstrual epilepsy

The charts of two epileptic patients, Margaret and Nancy, are shown in Figure 13; both responded completely to progesterone treatment and both had their driving licenses restored.

Rhinitis or *hayfever* is often mistaken for the *common cold.* It is usual to hear women in April saying "Do you know, this is the fourth cold I've had since Christmas" when in fact it is a premenstrual rhinitis occurring with the fourth menstruation since Christmas. Once it is recognized as a premenstrual symptom then the demand for antibiotics disappears. The rhinitis is due to extra water causing swelling of the cells of the nasal passages. If the swelling of the cells occurs a little lower down in the larynx it can cause *hoarseness*, which is a special nuisance to opera singers. One opera singer carefully arranged her singing engagements so that they avoided her premenstruum. Another remarked that during the premenstruum the quality of her voice changed and she was unable to reach the high notes. This was corrected by progesterone therapy.

The loss of a sense of smell is probably more common than generally appreciated and is presumably due to extra water accumulating in the cells responsible for the sense of smell. The manufacturer of a special brand of anti-perspirant/deodorant noticed that women tended to change their brand after three or four weeks use, complaining that it had ceased to function effectively. Market research showed that the dissatisfaction of the women was due to a premenstrual increase in sweating and vaginal discharge and a diminishing perception of the reassuring perfume of the anti-perspirant/deodorant product. This had led women falsely to believe that the product had lost its efficiency.

Dizziness or *vertigo* is a common complaint. In some surveys it occurred in a third of all sufferers of the premenstrual syndrome. It is most frequent among those who have had children and are approaching the menopause. The dizziness gets worse if she stoops and it may accompany a headache. The probable cause is excess fluid in the labyrinth of the ear, which is responsible for balance.

Similarly *fainting* is common just before menstruation, and is most likely to occur when there has been a long interval without food, or prolonged standing. It is common among teenage schoolgirls, who have missed their breakfast and have to stand for a long time at the early morning school assembly.

Cystitis and *urethritis* are common symptoms during the premenstruum and may be caused by the increase in vaginal discharge and generalized pelvic congestion.

Joint and *muscle pains* may come back each month just before menstruation, last only a few days and then disappear without treatment. There may also be stiffness on waking in the morning, although this disappears within the hour. The pain is likely to be due to localized swelling of the cells, or to the failure of muscle relaxation during the time of premenstrual tension. The presence of water retention in many of these symptoms led to the mistaken theory that the premenstrual syndrome was due to water retention, and could therefore be corrected by diurectics (water tablets). The effect of such treatment has already been discussed. (Pages 38–39)

There are many factors responsible for the formation of *varicose veins*, including a family tendency. However, when they first begin to appear they may only be visible in the premenstruum, later they may be painful only at this time of the cycle.

Boils, styes, herpes and *acne* are all common skin lesions which frequently come back each cycle just before menstruation. *Acne* is perhaps a special case. It is caused by the grease (or sebum) being too thick and too plentiful. This grease is produced by sebaceous glands in the skin and is excreted through the pores. If the grease is too thick it blocks the pores and causes acne. The skin only starts making grease, or sebum, at puberty, so in the first few years of its production there is often either too much or it is too thick or too thin. Gradually the body learns how to make the right amount. Estrogen helps to slow down the production of grease, so acne often comes back at the time of the falling estrogen level, such as at ovulation and before menstruation. This also explains why acne usually improves during pregnancy when there is plenty of estrogen, and also in some women who are on the high dosage estrogen pill.

Conjunctivitis, or red eye, may return each month due to causes other than infection. It is interesting that the association of conjunctivitis and menstruation was known as long ago as the sixteenth century.

Glaucoma is due to raised pressure within the eyeball. It can be caused by a narrowing of the opening through which the circulating fluid in the eyeball drains away, so it is not surprising to find that when there is water retention during the premenstruum there may be an excess accumulation of fluid within the eye and also difficulty in draining it away. (Figure 7) When this happens the pressure within the eye is raised, it becomes very painful and by pressure on the optic nerve may interfere with the sight. A survey of patients of menstruating age with closed angle glaucoma (where the draining opening is blocked) at the Institute of Ophthalmology, London, revealed that 89% suffered from the premenstrual syndrome. *Uveitis* and *iritis* are two other troublesome eye conditions which tend to flare up premenstrually and which respond so well to progesterone treatment.

Capricious appetite, food cravings and *binges* occurring at the height of premenstrual tension and water retention are well recognized. However great the self-control may be during the rest of the month, there come those days when she is "overtaken by a demon and eats enough for a week in just one meal."

Olive wrote:

"My life swings between cycles of feasting and fasting. Having lived on a careful diet of only 750 calories for two weeks and lost 4 lbs. I had an uncontrollable urge, which got me out of bed, raided mother's pantry and ate two loaves of bread with peanut butter, a packet of ginger cookies and an apple tart."

Doctors Smith and Sauder from McMaster University, Canada, studied three hundred nurses and confirmed the craving for food and sweets and the desire to eat compulsively during the times of premenstrual depression.

The actual foods chosen when there is a compulsive eating session are invariably carbohydrates and sweets, suggesting that the body's natural defense is coming into action to prevent a too severe or prolonged drop in blood sugar level (see pages 131–134).

Alcoholic bouts may be a feature of the paramenstruum. A survey of American female alcoholics revealed that 67% related it to the menstrual cycle and were able to abstain at other times; they all felt that their drinking habits had either started or increased during the premenstruum. During the paramenstruum the process of breaking down the alcohol appears to be slowed so that more accumulates in the blood stream. Many women find they cannot hold their normal amount of alcohol at this time, which is unfortunate as it implies that care is needed when taking alcohol as a pick-me-up to relieve the depression and tension.

Dentists recognize that *ulcers in the mouth* commonly recur during the premenstruum, and these are sometimes accompanied by ulcers in the vulva, vagina and anus. Most opticians have learned that when making appointments for fitting *contact lenses,* they must consider the time of the client's cycle for fitting may prove troublesome during the premenstruum. Similarly hairdressers know that if a permanent wave hasn't taken the chances are that it was done on the wrong day of the month.

Drug reactions are often reported during the premenstruum, and it always proves difficult to know exactly if it was due to the drug or a symptom of the premenstruum. This can also produce confusion when doctors are doing carefully controlled trials of new drugs. Often one finds the dummy tablet effective, whereas the real drug causes headaches, increased drowsiness or nausea. But it may be because the dummy tablet is being taken during the postmenstrual week when the woman is feeling well, and the real tablet during the premenstruum and she is just reporting her normal premenstrual symptoms.

Mention should also be made of pain known as the *Mittelschmerz*, or middle pain, which may occur at the time of ovulation. This is usually a mild cramping pain in the lower abdomen on one side or the other, usually alternating month by month. It is due to the release of the egg cell from the ovary and possibly to the contractions of the tubes as the egg cell makes its way down to the womb. The pain only lasts a few hours, and may be accompanied by a vaginal discharge or even slight bleeding. Young girls are apt to mistake it for acute appendicitis, and more than one teenager has arrived at my office complete with a packed case so that she could be sent straight off to hospital. In fact there is no vomiting, no distention of the abdomen and none of the usual signs of guarding and localization of pain which the doctors normally look for when they examine an abdomen. It is important to get these girls to record the time of abdominal pain as well as the dates of menstruation so that they themselves can appreciate the relationship. Although ovulation occurs alternately on the right or left side, it is not completely regular. For instance, it may be right, right, left, right, left, left, . . . so that at the end of the year it will probably have occurred an equal number of times on both sides.

7

Pain and Periods

A very welcome and much needed breeze of common sense has recently been wafted through the medical and gynecological fields by Drs. Jean and John Lennane, a husband and wife team who, in a well reasoned paper on a group of disorders which included period pain, point out that there is no justification for the old idea that "it is all in the mind" and that there is no real scientific evidence for such a claim. Indeed, all the scientific evidence that exists points to a hormonal imbalance. They use a number of quotations from current medical text books which they suggest have led to an irrational and ineffective approach to the treatment of such disorders. These quotations included the following:

> "It is generally acknowledged that this condition is much more frequent in the 'highly-strung,' nervous or neurotic female than in her more stable sister."

> "Faulty outlook . . . leading to an exaggeration of minor discomfort . . . may even be an excuse for not doing something that is disliked."

> "The pain is always secondary to an emotional problem."

> "Very little can be done for a patient who prefers to use menstrual symptoms as a monthly refuge from responsibility and effort."

The idea that period pains, or dysmenorrhea, are purely psychological was put forward because there were no abnormalities to be detected on full physical or gynecological examination, nor are there any suitable tests of hormone levels which can distinguish those who suffer once a month. However, gradually it is being realized that dysmenorrhea is due to an imbalance of hormones.

There are two quite different, and indeed opposite, types of dysmenorrhea, and as the treatment of the two types is different it is essential to distinguish between them. There is *spasmodic dysmenorrhea* which is characterized by spasms of abdominal pain, and *congestive dysmenorrhea* in which there is congestion of water or rather water retention. This latter type has all the characteristics of the premenstrual syndrome with the addition of period pains.

SPASMODIC DYSMENORRHEA

When menstruation first starts at puberty no ovulation occurs nor is there any period pain; however about two years later ovulation commences and then spasmodic dysmenorrhea also begins. Often at the beginning ovulation does not occur every month, but possibly only on alternate months, so period pains will only occur on alternate months. Spasmodic dysmenorrhea is most frequent between the ages of 15 and 25 years. It ends abruptly after a full term pregnancy, or it may gradually end with each period becoming less painful during the early twenties. The girl usually feels very well during the premenstruum and then is suddenly doubled up with severe spasms of pain in the lower abdomen on the first day of menstruation. The pain is colicky in nature, coming about every twenty minutes and lasting about five minutes, in fact they are similar to true labor pains. The girl obtains most relief by lying down curled up around a hot water bottle; aspirins may help take the edge off the pain, but gin is the old fashioned remedy. The pain may be so severe that bed is the only refuge, and pain may continue throughout the night preventing sleep. A monthly absence from work becomes the rule. The pain is easier on the second day and has passed by the third or fourth day. The distribution of pain is in the 'jock strap' area as shown in Figure 14, in fact it covers the area served by the uterine and ovarian nerves. The severity of the pain continues relentlessly month by month and is not affected by stress. It may be helped, temporarily at least, by an operation

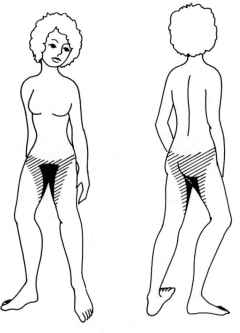

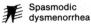 Spasmodic
dysmenorrhea

Figure 14   Site of pain in spasmodic dysmenorrhea

popularly known as a "D & C," or a dilation and curettage to stretch the opening of the womb. The girl is often immature with sparse hair in her armpits and lower abdomen, small breasts with pink nipples, and acne.

It would seem that spasmodic dysmenorrhea is due to insufficient estrogen for maturing and stretching the muscles of the womb. During pregnancy there is abundance of estrogen from the placenta for a full nine months, and also the muscle wall of the womb is stretched by the unborn babe, so after pregnancy this type of period pain ends and it is only on rare occasions that the woman subsequently suffers from the premenstrual syndrome, so there are some compensations.

Sufferers of spasmodic dysmenorrhea are often advised to take more exercise or alternatively to relax more. While doing a survey for the British consumer magazine "*Which?*" some years ago over two hundred women with spasmodic dysmenorrhea kept a careful record of the pain suffered for at least three cycles. It happened that the survey took place in the summer when many went on holiday. Some women normally had active jobs like waitress or nurses, and they tended to choose restful holidays lying in the sun. Others who had sedentary occupations chose active holidays, cycling 500 miles, mountaineering and surfing. However, regardless of their usual occupation or the amount of exercise they took, the amount of pain experienced was unaffected by the exercise or relaxation while on holiday.

A high level of another new hormone, called prostaglandin, has recently been found in sufferers from spasmodic dysmenorrhea; certain drugs known as prostaglandin inhibitors are most effective in relieving this type of pain.

CONGESTIVE DYSMENORRHEA

Congestive dysmenorrhea is the presence of heavy, continuous lower abdominal pain during the last seven days of the premenstruum, which increases in severity on the first day of menstruation and then gradually ceases, together with the end of the other premenstrual symptoms. The congestion was thought to be due to water retention. Congestive dysmenorrhea is another presentation of the premenstrual syndrome. In contrast to spasmodic dysmenorrhea, sufferers of the premenstrual syndrome may start with pain at their first menstruation and continue with it throughout their menstrual life, and the symptoms are present whether ovulation occurs or not. The pain is affected by stress, being worse when life in general is in a turmoil and being eased by happy events. A "D & C" brings no relief, nor does a pregnancy; in fact the premenstrual symptoms may be worse after each pregnancy. Again, in contrast to spasmodic dysmenorrhea, the sufferers of the premenstrual syndrome are more mature and maternal, with large breasts and brown nipples. An interesting fact is that smoking tends to enhance the pain in the premenstrual syndrome.

Estrogen administration increases the severity of the premenstrual syndrome, which responds to progesterone. Indeed excess progesterone administered to girls who have not borne children can cause spasmodic dysmenorrhea. Thus, in theory, either type of dysmenorrhea can be produced at will by overdosing with the wrong hormone, estrogen or progesterone, which in itself proves that painful periods are not psychological but are due to hormonal imbalance.

While stressing the benefit which can be obtained from appropriate treatment of painful periods, the very exceptional woman who does not ask for relief should not be forgotten. A 19-year-old filing clerk, living in a slum dwelling in a suburb in East London, was visited on one occasion for 'flu. In conversation her mother mentioned that she also suffered from severe period pains each month and would be brought home from the West End in a taxi. My immediate response was that suffering of this caliber was no longer necessary today, whereupon the girl replied "Oh don't! How else could I get a taxi ride once a month?"

MISPLACED CELLS

A rare cause of painful periods, which may come on with the first menstruation or after years of normal menstruation, and which affects only about one woman in twenty with dysmenorrhea, is due to a condition known as *endometriosis*. Cells of the lining of the cavity of the womb, or endometrium, become displaced, and may be found either in the muscle wall or outer coat of the womb itself, or in the ligaments around the womb, or ovary or anywhere in the lower abdomen. (Figure 15 shows the relative position of the organs around the womb.) These cells lining the cavity of the womb have a unique ability to multiply, be shed, grow again and multiply in an endless cycle under the menstrual hormonal influence. Each time the lining cells are shed they pass out from the opening of the womb, into the vagina and out of the body as a menstrual flow. However the misplaced cells are not able to shed out of the body, and instead tend to accumulate as tiny cysts which later become covered with scar tissue. Each time thickening of the lining occurs during the premenstruum these cysts become larger, and as the cells are shed at menstruation more room has to be found within these cysts for the extra cells, so you can well understand that after a time it becomes a very painful condition, with pain not limited only to the jock-strap area but spread all over the lower abdomen, possibly also affecting the bladder and rectum. In addition to the painful periods endometriosis is characterized by extreme pain during thrusting at intercourse, which may diminish and stop all sexual desire, and also by infertility due to scar tissue forming around the ovaries and tubes. Doctors can diagnose the condition by the story of painful periods, pain at intercourse and infertility, and also by gyne-

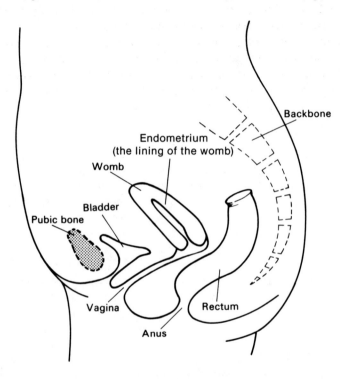

Endometrium
(the lining of the womb)

Backbone

Womb

Bladder

Pubic bone

Vagina

Rectum

Anus

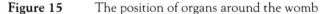

Figure 15　　The position of organs around the womb

cological examination and if necessary by laparascopy, an operation in which a minute periscope is inserted through a small cut in the abdominal wall and the surgeon can then see for himself the tiny cysts and surrounding scar tissue.

Why the cells become displaced remains a mystery. It is

possible that some were displaced during the developmental stage of the reproductive system in early fetal life, while it is also possible that some lining cells find their way through the fallopian tubes into the pelvis either at menstruation or labor. The pain is absent during pregnancy when there is no menstruation, although as already mentioned pregnancy does not often occur. The condition may be treated by stopping periods entirely for nine months or longer with hormone treatment. This not only stops menstruation, but also stops the cyclical changes in the normal and displaced endometrial cells.

8

Awkward Adolescent

The menarche, or first menstruation, is an important milestone in any girl's life and demonstrates that she has an intact hormonal pathway from the hypothalamus and pituitary to the ovaries and womb. It is heralded over a period of some two years by the development of secondary sex characteristics such as breast development, skin and circulatory changes, the growth of pubic and armpit hair and changes of the body shape into the rounded female figure. (Figure 16) However, it is not the end of pubertal development, and only represents about the halfway stage.

The changes in the breast occur very slowly, from the first development of a small 'bud' under the nipple the size of a grape, and gradually increasing in size to full development. Often one breast develops slightly before the other, but although this discrepancy often causes so much worry that immediate medical advice is sought, there is no cause for alarm. In due course both breasts will develop equally, for the growth stimulus comes from hormones in the bloodstream.

In India and Sri Lanka the first menstruation is a cause for celebration as it represents the girl's attainment of full maturity and the beginning of her sexual and reproductive life. The occasion is marked by a change from wearing short dresses to dressing in colorful and beautiful saris. There are reports that in Pakistan the girls in some households are deliberately fed on a low-protein diet in order to delay the menarche, thus postponing the cost of a marriage which is expected to occur immediately after the menarche has taken place.

The attitude taken towards this pubertal development depends very much on the culture of the society to which she belongs. In some societies such as Japan and Hong Kong, where the subject is still very taboo, the girls obtain their information furtively from the pages of the popular press. On the other hand in America today sex education is discussed so freely at home, at school and on the media that when the menarche occurs it is almost a non-event. The only girl in a male-dominated family may be especially fearful of the menarche, which emphasizes the many differences between herself and her brothers and may increase the conflict over her developing femininity.

The age of the menarche is influenced by racial, genetic, dietetic, social and economic factors. In Britain the average age of the menarche is 13.1 years, but it varies throughout the world being highest in the Bundi tribe in New Guinea at 18.8 years and lowest in Cuba at 12.4 years. There is an early menarcheal age among British children attending special schools for the deaf and blind where menarche occurs at the average age of 12.2 years, and even earlier menarcheal age among those with congenital abnormalities known to have started in early fetal life, like spina bifida and rubella. On the other hand the mentally disabled and those with Mongolism tend to have a later menarche. In Britain the range for normal children is from 10–16 years, in fact there is only one girl in a hundred who has not started menstruating by the age of 16 years. There has been a trend for the age of menarche to decrease since 1850, when it was 17.5 years; this decrease is attributed to better nutrition. It is thought that the age of menarche has stabilized in the last twenty-five years.

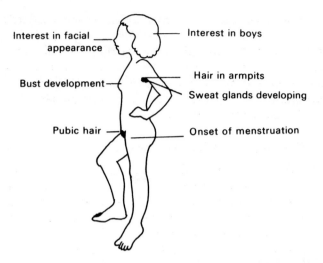

Figure 16   Development at puberty

The first menstruation usually lasts between three and eight days with an average of 5½ days, which is rather longer than most mothers expect it to be. There is then likely to be an interval of two or three months before the next menstruation. Only about four menstruations occur during the first year after the menarche, and gradually the cycle becomes shorter. Irregularity of periods is still quite frequent and at the age of 16 years 20% of girls still have cycles which last longer than 40 days, and 33% have a prolonged bleeding lasting at least seven days.

Irregularities of menstruation are quite common for teenagers and there are many quite normal reasons for this, but it can be very worrying for the girl herself. In these years she is not only adjusting to her developing feminine figure but she is also becoming more conscious of the opposite sex. As boyfriends come into the picture she becomes more interested in her own appearance, and these are often emotion-laden days.

In a single girl the cycle tends to be longer, perhaps 35 days, but as she begins to be stimulated by contact with boyfriends her cycle may shorten by a few days and reach nearer to the conventional norm, for the menstrual hormones are stimulated by male contact. However, if she is then jilted and returns to female companionship her cycle usually returns to its original pattern.

One 19-year-old inquired:

"My periods were always very irregular with sometimes even eight weeks between them. When I first met John they became better and once as short as 28 days. Then we had an awful quarrel and I broke up with him. Since then my cycles only seem to come when they want to, every five or six weeks. Does it matter?"

At nineteen it does not matter, and probably even before she received a reply she would have found another boyfriend and menstruation would have become more regular again.

About two years after the menarche, ovulation occurs, not necessarily every month initially but every two or three months, and gradually the cycles become more regular. It is with the onset of ovulation that spasmodic dysmenorrhea occurs. This usually comes as a surprise to both the girl and her mother as previously menstruation had been so painfree.

If spasmodic dysmenorrhea is bad enough to need regular medication to ease the pain, and especially if it causes the girl to take time off work or stay in bed, then medical help should be sought. It is interesting to listen to mothers explaining why they do not take their daughters to the doctor when they are suffering from spasmodic dysmenorrhea:

"I don't want to be considered fussy or neurotic."

"He will only tell her to get married and have children like I was told!"

"I would hate her to have an operation."

"He might put her on the pill; she's such a nice girl, besides she hasn't any boyfriends yet."

"Boys would take advantage of her if she were on the pill."

Such attitudes are a great shame as there is so much that can be done for these girls. If the parents do not want their daughter to have the pill the doctor can always prescribe estrogen alone, which is not contraceptive but will ease her monthly pains. However, since the introduction of prostaglandin inhibitors, estrogen and the pill are no longer the only effective treatment.

Even before the onset of the first menstruation cyclical mood swings are occurring, and they continue even at times of missed menstruation. (Figure 5) These mood swings can transform a happy schoolgirl into a lazy, bad-tempered, selfish individual whose academic work and behavior deteriorate even before menstruation is established. This is a story very suggestive of the premenstrual syndrome and events should be recorded so that help can be given to the girl before her work falls too far behind her schoolmates.

During these years one may anticipate marked conflicts between the early maturers and those who mature more slowly. Firm friendships of several years standing may be broken as one develops and "fancies herself as a lady" and the other remains a mere schoolgirl. With maturation comes the interest in boys and an appreciation of feminine beauty, so that endless time is spent in caring for her face and body. At this time grease starts developing in the skin and the sweat glands begin to operate, so that skin care and deodorants become necessary.

Many girls do not like the changes in body contour which Nature has decreed; they object to the rounded contours and would prefer the broad shoulders and gawky limbs of boys. This stimulates the urge to diet, particularly in those who are not even overweight for their height and size. Excessive dieting during these developing years may halt menstruation and ovulation and lead to *anorexia nervosa*. It is not unusual to find girls reducing their weight by strict dieting from 120 lbs. to 70 lbs. within a few months, and yet still complaining of their body-image and imagining that they are too fat. Unhappily the road to recovery in such cases is slow and halting, and their future fertility is at stake, indeed when menstruation does return it is often accompanied by unpleasant premenstrual symptoms.

Unfortunately for most teenagers this sexual development is occurring just at the same time as their mothers are experiencing the difficult years of the menopause and are also subject to mood swings and unpleasant symptoms. Nevertheless it is important to help adolescents through this stage, however awkward, impossible and thoughtless they become. They should be given every opportunity to mix freely with both older girls and children, and with boys and men, to help them sort themselves out and appreciate the differences in individual men and women.

At puberty it is the premenstrual depression which is usually worse than the tiredness, and is likely to make a girl sullen, secretive, withdrawn and anxious to be alone. Nevertheless careful observation should be kept of her behavior, as too often the mood swings occur suddenly without warning or provocation and she may make an unexpected suicide gesture.

Phyllis, 17 years old, had been at the top of her class at 12 years old, and her work was the envy of others. But she gradually went downhill in work and behavior. She became slovenly, rude and bored with everything, gave up any attempt at graduating from high school and left school at the first opportunity. She first worked in a hairdresser's shop, but her work was unsatisfactory and her time-keeping poor. Her next job was as a filing clerk, where her work was not appreciated. There would be days when she would come home, slip up to her bedroom and stay there for hours, allowing no one to enter and refusing food. One day her father found her apparently asleep in a corner, but the doctor diagnosed an overdose of hypnotics and arranged for her admission to hospital for a stomach wash-out. This incident so shocked her mother that from then onwards she kept a careful eye on her daughter. Soon the mother noted the correlation of awkwardness and menstruation and asked for medical help. With treatment her daughter brightened up again, restarted her social life which had been absent for five years and later returned to evening classes obtaining higher qualifications in shorthand and typing.

Girls with the premenstrual syndrome deserve treatment in their teens, and usually the need for progesterone is only temporary. Gradually as they mature the need for regular medication passes, although they may need it again in times of stress.

At one British boarding school parents and visitors were invited to inspect the dormitories on the annual Open Day. On the mantelpiece in each of the spotless dormitories was displayed a grade sheet giving the grade each child had received for the tidiness of her bed and locker before going down to breakfast each morning. It was not difficult on inspecting these sheets to determine the menstrual patterns of the girls, for when they were exceptionally sleepy during the premenstruum they were more likely to receive a poor tidiness grade.

At another boarding school, punishment books were used for recording the names of girls, the date and the reasons for the punishments. These books were made available for analysis together with the books the girls signed when they menstruated and needed sanitary protection. It was found that during menstruation the girls were twice as naughty as would have been expected. Many of the punishments during menstruation were those which could be accounted for by tiredness, and included such offences as forgetfulness and unpunctuality, while others reflected the premenstrual irritability at having to conform to strict school discipline. Indeed a girl is more likely to be punished for any offence during menstruation as she may be too slow to avoid detection. If several children are all talking when the teacher enters the classroom, it will be those with a slow reaction time who will not stop talking quickly enough and will receive a punishment.

This investigation also showed two types of naughtiness. When it had been completed the principal, an exceptional woman who knew and was concerned with each individual girl, was shown two lists of girls' names and asked to comment on them. Unknown to her the lists contained the names of the girls who had received most punishments during the term. One list contained the names of those whose punishments had all occurred during the premenstruum. "Just naughty girls from exuberance or laziness; I'll probably be choosing a future head girl from that list," she commented. But when shown the other list containing the names of girls whose punishments had occurred evenly throughout the menstrual cycle she remarked, "They're the problem girls requiring careful handling and understanding," and she went on to describe how they had to cope with such difficulties as broken homes, foreign parents, or minor deformities such as a harelip.

In the study it was also noted that teachers' helpers,

girls of 16–18 who were permitted to punish girls for misbehavior, gave significantly more punishments during their own menstruations, and then their standard gradually fell throughout the cycle. This naturally raises the problem of the teachers, and indeed any woman in charge, such as magistrates and forewomen: do they give more punishments during their own menstruation? Are they more strict then? Or, once they appreciate the effect of menstrual hormones on their behavior, do they lean over backwards to try to avoid punishing too severely when they themselves are menstruating?

In this survey it was also possible to analyze how many days passed before a girl who had been punished once was punished a second time, a statistical method known as "critical-event analysis." The results showed that most second punishments occurred within four days of the first offence, then less within five to eight days of the first offence, and so there was a gradual decrease in further punishments until 25–28 days after the first offence when there was an unexpected rise not only in those girls who were already menstruating but also in girls who had not yet started. This suggests that already these premenarche girls were experiencing mood swings, a fact that many observant mothers have already noticed in their daughters. Incidentally it was possible to do a similar analysis in respect of boys at the nearby boarding school, but they did not show evidence of cyclical mood swings.

On one occasion my adolescent daughter burst into the house from school asking for a menstrual chart. When asked why, she replied that her teacher had lost her temper and thrown a piece of chalk at a girl, and the same thing had occurred on the Thursday before semester break which was exactly four weeks earlier!

When my daughter left the twelfth grade she passed on to the next head girl of the school a list, compiled by the girls, of the probable dates of the teachers' menstruations so that the girls would know when to hand in their essays to get good grades.

When, in later years, schoolgirls meet and exchange memories it is the unfair incidents and unjustified punishments which are uppermost in their minds. One now wonders how often the blame could have been placed on it being the wrong day of the month for the teachers.

School principals have a dual responsibility: not only to cope with their own premenstrual mood swings, but also to recognize the existence of them in the girls for whose education they are responsible. They should be ready to step in with a kind word to girls who appear to have episodes of irritability or become depressed or disheartened, giving encouragement, particularly in preventing a girl from giving up a worthwhile career just because of some minor pinpricks or temporary difficulties of study.

Schoolgirls' work deteriorates during the premenstruum. (Figure 6) A similar survey of girls in the Armed Forces confirmed lower intelligence scores in tests performed by the girls during the paramenstruum.

A study into the effect of menstruation on the results of high school and college level examinations showed that those girls taking examinations during the paramenstruum had fewer passes, less distinction grades and a lower average grade. The girls whose results were most affected during the paramenstruum were those with cycles exceeding 31 days, and those whose menstruation lasted for seven days or longer. In the high school examinations, some subjects were completed in one day, some had tests four days apart and other subjects had tests at an interval of more than eight days. Consideration of the results in relation to the time intervals between exams on the same subject showed that girls were under greater handicap in those subjects where all tests were completed in one day, (when she could be in her paramenstruum) in comparison to subjects where exams were spaced more than eight days apart, in which case the girl could not have been entirely in her paramenstruum during both exams. It should not be difficult for examination boards and universities so to arrange examination timetables that when two tests are necessary for a subject they are eight or more days apart.

It might be mentioned that at public examinations provision is usually made for proctors to make a note at the top of the examination paper of candidates who are handicapped by the paramenstruum at the time of writing the exam. But it is not known how much notice is taken of this fact by the examiners.

Another hazard is the increased sex desire which may occur premenstrually. This often takes over young adolescents, who are quite unprepared for this new sex urge, and unable to control their emotions. This nymphomanic urge may be responsible for young girls running away from home or custody, only to be found wandering in the park or following boys. These girls can be helped and their delinquent behaviour abruptly ended with progesterone therapy.

9

Marriage

One wonders whether the cynic who wrote: "Marriages are made in heaven, but they end up in hell!" was married to a wife who was a severe case of the premenstrual syndrome, or was he just a keen observer of other people's marriages. Of course, not all marriages end up in hell, but for the young groom whose bride suffers from the premenstrual syndrome or later develops it, the stakes run pretty high. Most men enter marriage sublimely ignorant of the problems women face each month; such knowledge as they have is probably confined to a vague awareness of "the monthlies" when she bleeds and is "on the rag." If their mothers or their sisters were sufferers they might have learned how to cope with it, but the odds are that they are inclined to think that they were unique in their troubles and really know little about the cause.

Before marriage, and whilst they were going out together, it was easy enough for the girl to conceal those difficult days and all too often it is not until they are living together that the awful truth begins to dawn. If she is a sufferer from spasmodic dysmenorrhea he will be the first to see that she gets good and complete relief of her pains, for pain is something a man can understand. However, sudden mood changes, irrational behavior, and bursting into tears for no apparent reason are bewildering, while sudden aggression and violence are deeply disturbing when, with little warning and no justification, his darling little love bird suddenly becomes an angry, argumentative, shouting, abusive bitch.

Fortunately, not all women suffer from the premenstrual syndrome, nor do all premenstrual syndrome sufferers become hellcats. Even so the groom-to-be should be made aware of the problem that can arise, how to recognize it when it first shows itself and what treatment is available to provide complete relief. An article in *Bride and Home* described what may lie ahead for the husband once the honeymoon is over:

> "Then quite suddenly you feel as if you can't cope any more – everything seems too much trouble, the endless household chores, the everlasting planning of meals. For no apparent reason you rebel: 'Why should I do everything?' you ask yourself defiantly. 'I didn't have to do this before I was married. Why should I do it now?' Everything starts going wrong and it gets worse instead of better.
>
> As on other mornings you get up and cook breakfast while your husband is in the bathroom. You climb wearily out of bed and trudge down the stairs, a vague feeling of resentment growing within you. The sound of cheerful whistling from upstairs only makes you feel a little more cross. Without any warning the toast starts to scorch and the sausages instead of happily sizzling in the pan start spitting and spluttering furiously. Aghast you rescue the toast which by this time is beyond resurrection and fit only for the trash. The sausages are charred relics of their former selves and you throw those out too. Your unsuspecting husband opens the kitchen door expecting to find his breakfast ready and waiting, only to see a smoky atmosphere and a thoroughly overwrought wife. You are so dismayed at him finding you in such chaos that you just burst helplessly into tears."

What is the young husband going to make of that situation? Much depends upon his family background. If he has met similar situations in his home before marriage he will undoubtedly react as he did then, so that if he used to make himself scarce and get out of the house, he'll probably grab his bag and dash for the office leaving her to sort out her troubles. If he was in the habit of helping to sort out the chaos, he'll probably sympathize with her, give her a kiss, and make her a cup of coffee and breakfast and insist on her going back to bed for the day. This latter is the wisest course of action.

But what if the young husband has never met this sort of thing. How will he cope? Will he shrug it off hoping that it is only a temporary lapse until, once a month, month after month it recurs? Or will he rage about breakfast being ruined and storm out of the house to arrive at work hungry and unable to do his work properly? Eventually returning home in a tired and frustrated state to an equally distraught wife? Not a happy augury for the future.

So far, in this chapter, we've been considering the state of the premenstrual syndrome bride. There are those who don't start their symptoms until after a pregnancy. Just think of the situation. For a year or more they've been enjoying an idyllic married life until the baby comes along and now once a month there are the frustrations, mood swings, irritability and apparent laziness in addition to coping with the baby. From being the "blue-eyed boy" he now finds that he can do nothing right on those terrible days. If he has been a sensible husband and kept a diary of her menstrual dates he will soon recognize the time relationship and, being sensible, will insist on her seeing a doctor and obtaining treatment for her premenstrual syndrome.

On the other hand if he hasn't been sensible, if neither he nor she has any clear idea of her menstrual dates they'll probably go on month after month until he can stand it no longer.

But all this suffering is quite unnecessary and a tragic destruction of family life. The answer to it lies in the true nature of marriage, which is that bride and groom, husband and wife share equally in every aspect of their lives. If, when they are engaged, they both keep a chart of her menstruation and any symptoms that she may have, they will soon realize when things are going wrong and then is the time to seek medical advice and obtain treatment for it. If together they keep the chart it will help them to understand each other better and the fiancé, and later husband, will have a much greater understanding of what menstruation means to a woman. He will also find that he is the first to notice the warning signs of the premenstrual syndrome. The slight irrationality of her conversation, or lack of conversation, the minor disagreements in which there is a certain rigidity in her views. More important still is the darkening of the skin around the eyes, one of the surest signs that she is about to enter her premenstruum. In some women the skin goes so dark as to appear almost black.

If at this time the fiancé or husband suggests that she should start her treatment, or go to the doctor he will receive a flat denial that there is anything wrong. In fact she is quite unaware of the changes taking place, but this rigid refusal is another sure sign. If they have together been keeping a chart of her menstruation this is the time to bring it out and check together the timing, when the time relationship should be confirmed. If she is already on progesterone therapy, the husband can then insist that she starts using her progesterone suppositories or takes some extra, or if she is not undergoing treatment he should take her along to the doctor together with the menstrual chart, or to a Premenstrual Syndrome Clinic if one is available. If treatment is not started at once, within 2–3 days she will be in the midst of her symptoms and it is then difficult to do much to help, for once the symptoms are there progesterone will not work.

Progesterone must always be given before the symptoms start. All the husband can do is to offer her sympathy and assure her that he loves her, all of which will probably be rejected, but he must persist.

If there are children he should remember that they are more likely to get out of hand with mother no longer able to care for and play with them. He must try to be a substitute mother as well as a father and exercise his control over them. He should remember that there is housework to be done and it is no use telling her to rest, he has to be practical. If the work has to be done and there is no one else to do it, she will not rest. A neighbor or a relative could be asked to help, it will probably only be for four or five days, unless it is very severe. Once menstruation has started and while events are still fresh in their minds he should impress upon her the need for medical help and assure her that he will go with her. More husbands accompany their wives to the doctor or hospital when asking help for the premenstrual syndrome than for any other gynecological condition, and this includes the infertile couples seeking help.

The following quotes from recent mail reveal how often the husband is implicated in the premenstrual syndrome:

"I am fortunate in having an extremely long-suffering husband who puts up with my tirades as best he knows how, but he says he doesn't know how to cope with me."

"My husband first noticed the connection with my menstrual cycle without mentioning it to me eighteen months ago, and backs me up completely in writing to you."

"The misery has gone on for years, misery and misery. Seventeen jobs in ten years. Now I clean offices, and for two weeks out of the month my husband gets up at 4:00 A.M. and does them for me."

Not uncommonly the husbands have devised their own means of confirming the diagnosis beforehand, thus the computer magnate came complete with a computer print-out to prove it, while a draughtsman turned up with a beautifully drawn blueprint, others merely bring along the office diary or kitchen calendar.

But there are still too many husbands who have not made the diagnosis, or more rarely do not realize that help is available. They may know when they wake up that it's one of those days and, no matter what they do, they will not be able to satisfy their wife. If he returns home with some red roses she'll ask "Why didn't you bring me my favorite chocolates?," but when he brings the correct brand of chocolates it'll be "You know I'm dieting, how very cruel of you." He just can't win.

The monthly problems may interfere with his social life and his earning capacity. Some years ago a door-to-door salesman was sent by his employer for medical help. He worked on a commission basis, and while his average weekly takings were quite high, in one week in four the sum fell to something much lower. Not only did he find it difficult to plan to make ends meet financially, but his chances of promotion were affected. The salesman explained that he became more depressed and seemed to start work later during the weeks his earnings were low. When asked about his wife's menstruation the significance gradually dawned on him. A few days later he brought along his wife's menstrual record which confirmed the diagnosis. Her irritability and tiredness were hindering her husband. She was delighted to be offered progesterone treatment and responded well. Her husband was also delighted when he got a promotion.

Marital disharmony is a recurring theme among those seeking medical help:

"My marriage broke up seven years ago and I feel this trouble was a big cause of the break-up. I have since turned down a chance to remarry as I cannot face burdening someone with my continual monthly ailments."

"This premenstrual misery is a very real threat to the survival of our marriage."

"We have been married for eight years during which time my premenstrual tension has been a constant problem. During the past three years this has become more acute and increasingly more severe with a traumatic effect on our relationship and that with our two boys of five and three years."

"My husband has urged me to write, our marriage is breaking up, my children are suffering and after five years of my trouble my poor husband can take no more."

"My husband has already left me and I have two children who I try hard not to lose my temper with at this time, but I feel sorry for them, it is really awful."

"I have come to dread my periods and even my husband rushes to the calendar at an unexpected outburst on my part. I get violent with my husband."

Sometimes the marital disharmony is just silence, on other occasions there are vicious verbal battles, and at the extreme limit there are the fights and batterings. How many wives batter their husbands during their paramenstruum is unknown, nor do we know how often the husband is provoked beyond endurance and batters her.

One mother wrote about her daughter who was receiving treatment for premenstrual irritability and food cravings:

"Some cakes and cookies disappeared on Sunday. It was all too much for me and I burst into tears. This in turn upset my husband who went and found Mary in her bedroom and gave her a good thrashing. At midnight we discovered she was missing. She had spent the night with friends. Both Mary and I started menstruating that day."

Here is a case of menstrual synchrony, with mother's and daughter's menstruation occurring at the same time and where the mother's tears caused the fraught husband to beat his daughter.

Two researchers in Washington, D.C., Roger Langley and Richard Levy, have estimated that there are 12 million battered husbands in the United States. They reckon it is the "most unreported crime," affecting 20% of husbands. Again one is just left wondering on the effect of the para-menstruum, how often were the wives also victims of their own hormonal imbalance?

A couple of quotes to suggest that the premenstruum may frequently be the cause:

"I attacked him with a carving knife on one occasion, and whilst building a stone wall I lifted huge stones and hurled them at him."

"I have tried to knife my husband too many times to count . . . but for one fantastic week I feel on top of the world."

Most marriage-guidance counselors are well versed in the traumas which can be caused to the marital relationship by the premenstrual syndrome and try to draw the partner's attention to this. The wise counselors, when telephoned urgently for help because of a massive quarrel, will arrange a meeting seven days later when the woman is more likely to be in her rational postmenstrual phase, having more insight and being more amenable to reason.

While the wife may be content for most of the month coping with the cooking, cleaning, shopping, mending, ironing, and perhaps even the gardening, there may come one of those days when it all gets on top of her, when she's too apathetic to cope with everyday chores, when she burns the cooking, and leaves the house untidy and in a slovenly condition. Alternatively she may have a spurt of restless energy, obsessionally polishing all and sundry until she wears herself out and then blames her premenstrual symptoms on the fact that she "overdid it." One difficulty facing the housewife at home all day is the temptation to miss meals, waiting to enjoy an evening meal with her husband at night. During the paramenstruum she will be facing the problems of low blood sugar levels.

The working wife faces different problems. In her effort to control herself in front of her workmates, and possibly also the public, she stores up her problems until she reaches home and then lets go at her nearest and dearest. Again she may well have missed her lunch and gone a long interval without food not appreciating the problems this causes.

A most important problem the couple must face will be that of sexual harmony. Dr. Ruth D'arcy Hart, Medical Officer at the Fertility and Problems Clinic in London, found that among married women 60% noted their sex urge was greatest before menstruation, but unfortunately for those with the premenstrual syndrome this is also the time at which many of them are most horrible to their husbands, and when to spite him they refuse his sexual overtures. It is the time when it is so easy for her to claim she's too tired. Incidentally one of the side effects of the pill, too rarely mentioned, is its ability to decrease the natural sex urge. Satisfactory sex between partners is the best cement for any marriage. There is so much that can be done these days, if difficulties develop in this side of marriage, that it is worthwhile seeking help. One cause of a decrease in sexual satisfaction, which has only recently been recognized but is most responsive to treatment, is a loss of sex urge occurring after a pregnancy complicated by postnatal depression. A blood test may show the wife to have a raised prolaction level, in which case treatment with bromocriptine can be effective.

Men do not have cycles akin to women. On page 76 a "critical event analysis" is described which detected cycles of naughtiness in premenarcheal girls. A similar one has also been done in various surveys of men and women in relation to prisoners, schoolboys and symptoms of glaucoma. The results were similar except that there appeared to be a return of the critical event after an interval of 25–28 days in women but not in men.

Margaret Henderson of Australia has shown that men have a similar ovulation temperature chart which is synchronous with the wife's chart. When the wife has a mid-cycle temperature drop followed by a rise at ovulation, which then continues at a higher level until menstruation, the husband also has the sudden drop in temperature followed by a rise, but the temperature does not then stay up continuously. However, if the wife has an anovular cycle with no drop and rise at ovulation, the husband's chart follows suit and he does not have an ovular rise. If the wife goes on the pill or becomes pregnant, and so stops ovulating, again the husband does not have the characteristic drop and rise. If the man moves out to live alone or with another man, again the characteristic drop and rise will be lost. All of which suggests that when a couple are in harmony together their body's rhythm is synchronous, the man taking the lead from the woman's cycle.

As mentioned earlier a good proportion of husbands will attend at the doctor's office with the wife if she is suffering from the premenstrual syndrome, and the remainder will usually agree to come together at the next interview.

This is a most valuable opportunity to learn more of the full extent of the wife's problems. At the same time there is much useful information which can be given to the husband to help him cope better with the situation. First, he must understand what the premenstrual syndrome is and why it occurs, and should appreciate which of his wife's symptoms can be helped and which are not premenstrual but occurring throughout the month, and therefore not likely to benefit from progesterone treatment. He should be taught how to chart the symptoms, and may like to keep his own chart of events. Often the husband is the first to appreciate that his wife could benefit by some extra progesterone, and if she is receiving it by suppositories it is usually possible to give him full permission to raise the dose when he feels the need is there. The husband should also appreciate the problems of low blood sugar levels, and that his wife will be worse if deprived of sleep. He should also appreciate that at times of water retention her alcohol consumption should be reduced.

If the husband fully understands the situation he will be able to make the necessary adjustments to their life. Thus one husband, realizing his wife's irritability in the premenstruum, asked the bank manager to send their joint balance sheets on specified days so that they could discuss their financial arrangements calmly in her postmenstruum. During the premenstruum when the wife has little insight many decisions like moving, holidays and schools must either be taken by the husband or postponed for a week or so until rational discussions are a possibility. If help in the home is needed it may be better to arrange this for the one vital week of the month rather than merely one day per week.

10

Mother

The mother is the lynchpin of the family. When her life becomes a misery each month, because of the disturbances of the premenstrual syndrome, the consequences affect the whole family: husband, babies, schoolchildren and teenagers. Children, even infants of only a few months, are sensitive to changes in mother's temperament, and because they cannot understand the reason, they react to it in their own peculiar way.

When you ask adult sufferers of the premenstrual syndrome if their mother also suffered in the same way you are likely to get many positive, and some interesting, replies, such as:

"We used to say 'The dragon's on the warpath' and we all knew what it meant. But it only lasted a day or two."

"I remember my brother putting up a red flag outside the front door to warn us to be careful in our approach to mother."

Health visitors and social workers soon recognize when one of the mothers in their care is in her premenstruum. The usually tidy house is slovenly and disorganized, the carpets littered with old clothes, dirty dishes still on the kitchen table and probably a burnt cake by the sink. Maybe the children went off to school late, and in yesterday's clothes, and the chances are that the meals will not be ready on time.

Although the premenstrual syndrome may start at puberty it usually gets worse – or it can begin – after the children are born, especially if there has been any depression after childbirth. This was a recurring theme in many letters:

"Since the birth of my last child two years ago (I have five children) I have changed from being a perfectly normal housewife and mother to an unpredictable bad-tempered person. During my period my moods make me feel positively ill, especially my head. If only I could grow a new one, I say to my husband."

"I have had intervals of depression since the birth of my first child so that I have never regained confidence in myself since then."

"After baby's birth I changed and now I get an incredible amount of head pressure for a few days prior to the bleeding. It was as though the top of my head was about to blow off with pressure. I spoke to my doctor about the possibility of me starting an early menopause, but he only smiled and said it was more likely premenstrual tension."

"I have a twenty-two-month-old son and I cannot remember feeling like this before he was born. I do love him very much but the poor little soul does have a terrible time when I shout at him and make him sob his heart out and I seem unable to stop although I feel terrible about what I'm doing. It is almost as though I must be getting some sort of pleasure from it, and I feel very, very upset and guilty afterwards."

Dr. Christine Cooper, a pediatrician, has stated that children can also be psychologically damaged for life by verbal violence.

The sudden onset of irritability after the birth of a child is a cause of surprise to many mothers, who did not experience it before. They suddenly find themselves becoming quick-tempered, and making totally irrational decisions. They become impatient with the children, not waiting for them to learn to dress or eat for themselves. They won't accept that "kids will be kids" and shout at them when they are romping about harmlessly and then complain that the children won't behave. They are like the schoolteacher's helpers who expect a higher standard of discipline when they themselves are menstruating.

When mother's got so much to do it's easy enough to miss out on meals, which always has the additional benefit of slimming too. Unfortunately her irritable and aggressive outbursts are likely to occur when her blood sugar level is at its lowest which makes matters even worse.

Rose, an intelligent unmarried mother of 24 years, had contacted the National Society for the Prevention of Cruelty to Children herself as she feared she might harm her six-year-old son during her premenstruum. It was obvious from her story that she had been very near to damaging him. She then described the usual timetable for the day, "getting up at 8:00 A.M. and having a meal of toast and coffee together and then walking half a mile to his school, doing the shopping on the way home, housework until it was time to fetch him from school at 3:30 P.M." This was the worst time of the day and just before her periods she would feel aggressive as she met him, suddenly a surge of hatred would well up and if he didn't behave, this is the time he would be smacked.

In fact Rose was describing how she became irritable with her son 7½ hours after her last meal, having been energetic during the interval. Her menstrual chart confirmed that she only lost her temper during the premenstruum, and since having treatment with progesterone and eating a midday meal she has been happier and trouble-free. Incidentally she would mark in advance on her menstrual chart the days on which she had to exert extra self-control as she was so anxious to do all that was best for her son.

Two remarks often heard after successful treatment of these patients are "Even my children behave better" and "They don't shout so much nowadays."

Contraception often proves a problem for these mothers. Those with the premenstrual syndrome are liable to have side effects on the pill. Intrauterine devices can cause increased estrogen production, resulting in heavy menstruation becoming even heavier. Unfortunately tubal ligation, previously thought to be a convenient permanent solution, has been shown to reduce the progesterone blood level. If they are receiving progesterone this can be used contraceptively, as discussed on page 187.

CHILDREN CANNOT UNDERSTAND

Children, who cannot understand the mood swings in their mothers, may react with the development of psychosomatic or bodily symptoms, such as a cough, running nose, endless crying, temper tantrums or vomiting. In my general practice when children attended with such complaints the mother would be given a chart on which to record the dates of the child's symptoms and another one for mother to record the dates of her own menstruation. When the mother returned with the charts after an interval of two or three months it was surprizing how often it was clearly shown that the child was reacting, with various ailments, to mother's mood swings. A survey of 100 mothers visiting the doctor because their child had a cough or cold showed that 54% of the mothers were in their paramenstruum. The children who were brought during the mother's paramenstruum had a tendency to be under two years, only children, those with symptoms of less than 24-hours duration and those whose mothers were under 30 years of age. One girl was only nine months, yet her mother brought a chart showing that for the previous three months each time she had menstruated the child had developed a cough and runny nose.

A six-month-old girl was brought to the office with herpes (or shingles) on her knee, by her mother who had recurrent premenstrual herpes on her upper lip of several years duration.

A further survey was carried out among children who were admitted as emergencies to the North Middlesex Hospital in London. The mothers of 100 children were interviewed, and the result was very similar, in fact 49% of the mothers were in their paramenstruum on the day the child was admitted. Some were admitted because of an illness such as asthma, abdominal pain, or a temperature of unknown cause, while others had been injured in an accident. If the mother is accident prone during her paramenstruum, the child she is looking after is also accident prone. If mother is tired during the paramenstruum she will not notice little Johnny running into an oncoming car or climbing a dangerous tree, and so even he will be in greater danger then.

One day a telephone call informed me that an 18-month-old boy had had a high temperature and a convulsion. This was the third convulsion at intervals of three to four weeks. Enquiry revealed that it was not related to mother's menstrual cycle, but to the Nanny, who had total care of the boy while his mother worked full-time. There had been some trouble with Nanny the day before and she had just been given notice. The two previous convulsions had occurred at the time of Nanny's para-menstruum.

SIBLING JEALOUSY

Sometimes jealousy of a brother or sister is incorrectly diagnosed, when the real diagnosis is the premenstrual syndrome in the mother.

Susan, aged 30 years, had been very well during her second pregnancy, with plenty of energy so that she would take three-year-old David out each afternoon to play on the swings or kick a football in the nearby recreation park. She had an easy delivery of a much-wanted daughter, but afterwards became so depressed that she needed psychiatric treatment. David had been dry since the age of sixteen months, but after his sister's birth he gradually started to wet the bed again, not every night, but in batches every few weeks. It seemed all too easy to blame it onto jealousy of the new baby, but when the mother kept a careful record it showed that David's bedwetting was occurring during mother's premenstruum. Mother then agreed she "hadn't been the same" since the baby's birth, and had been too tired and busy to take David out for his usual playtime in the park.

BATTERED CHILDREN

The most tragic presentation of the premenstrual syndrome is when it reaches such severity that the mother, in a state of confusion and rage, batters her much-loved child. These mothers, contrary to popular belief, are women who really love their child, they have strong maternal feelings, but in a sudden moment of premenstrual irritability their control is lost and they injure their darling child.

A social worker's report on a 35-year-old mother of two children reads:

> "During the last premenstruum her youngest daughter, aged 18 months, was screaming and would not stop. Patient was very irritated by this and picked her up and squeezed her – this started a circle of louder screaming and harder squeezing until patient 'heard something crack.' She was immediately frightened and threw the child on the floor and sat crying on the chair. When more composed she examined Joan and took her to the doctor."

This type of injury to a child is not uncommon. Judging by the letters and confidences of patients, it suggests that the cases of baby-battering that are coming to light are only the tip of an iceberg.

> "Because I lost my temper and hit my eldest child when he was four, just before a period, I nearly had a complete nervous breakdown. Even though I feel much better now my premenstrual tension remains and from day 18 of the cycle until day 4 of my period I suffer from depression, temper, forgetfulness and dizziness."

> "It has got to a stage now that every month something

the children do triggers me off. It is as though there is somebody inside saying terrible things. I blame my son and tell him I hate him and hit him. Sometimes he gets out of my way quickly."

If the situation deteriorates the children may be taken into care, but this is a drastic step. One is left wondering about the after-effects on the many slightly battered children, those who are not spotted by the social services and are not helped. Does the unsettled temperamental background of childhood leave any marks such as shyness or lack of confidence?

A woman who had been treated with progesterone for seventeen years was asked if she would like to take part in a television commentary dealing with the premenstrual syndrome. She went home and explained to her family that she couldn't recall those far-off days, "By Jove – Dad and I will never be able to forget your vicious temper" was the comment by the daughter, now in her twenties.

A 35-year-old teacher married to a principal stated:

"For seven days during the premenstruum I become tense, irritable, shouting, weepy and tired, bloated with swelling of my legs and ankles and with headaches over my eyes. I have two children and at those times when I am in an uncontrollable temper I have hit them really hard."

She was successfully treated with progesterone for twelve months and has been free from symptoms since. She later wrote:

"It has been a valuable experience – I would never have believed that an intelligent woman like me, with high morals and good education, could ever lose control of herself to such an extent that she would batter her children, for I love my children dearly. How utterly illogical it is that I personally should cause them permanent harm."

When the child reaches school the teacher may notice that absences seem to be occurring at regular intervals. One ten-year-old girl was referred for treatment by her teacher who noticed absences for a few days at the beginning of each month. The teacher, in fact, wondered if it was because of the girl's menstruation, but it transpired that mother had recurrent premenstrual asthma requiring rest in bed and the daughter was kept at home to answer the door.

TEENAGERS' REACTIONS

Playing truant from school may also occur, as in the case of one mother who wrote:

"For days before a period starts I hate everyone and make the family's life a misery. My thirteen-year-old daughter will not go to school when I'm like this. She is frightened of what I will do and cries when I start drinking."

Teenagers, both boys and girls, are quick enough to spot the changes in their mother and notice when she's "in one of those moods" or as one boy said "our whole life revolves around Mom's periods."

The mother's problem is not helped when the daughter starts to menstruate if they both occur together in synchrony. Many mothers, recognizing the problem in themselves, initially seek help for their daughter's premenstrual syndrome, believing that as they've weathered the storm so far it won't be long before the end. However, they are not prepared to let their daughters suffer as they have done.

Finally all mothers, and fathers too, have the responsibility of seeing that their children get good sex education, and especially know about those problems which come back once a month.

11

The World's Workers

The cost to industry of menstrual problems is high, and it is measured in millions of pounds, liras, kroners or dollars, not in terms of human misery, unhappiness or pain. It has been estimated to cost British industry 3% of its total wage bill, which may be compared with 3% in Italy, 5% in Sweden and 8% in America. The load is not spread evenly, for the industries which suffer most are those employing large numbers of women, especially the clothing industry, light-engineering, transistor and assembly factories and laundries. Texas Instruments, which employs women for the assembly of electrical components, finds that the average worker's normal production rate of 100 components per hour drops during the paramenstruum to 75 per hour.

Research studies have shown that during the paramenstruum there is a deterioration of arm and hand steadiness, which is an adverse factor among those whose work demands manual dexterity. One podiatrist complained that during the paramenstruum her hands get stiff and she finds skilled movements difficult. "If ever I do cut a patient you can be sure it will be during those premenstrual days." One wonders if the same ever applies to surgeons.

Absenteeism, directly from menstrual problems, is generally due to spasmodic dysmenorrhea, premenstrual migraine and asthma for, as one library assistant remarked, "you don't stay away from work merely because of your bad temper, instead you soldier on and cause chaos by misfiling, and you get yourself a bad name." The influence of menstrual illness during working hours was demonstrated in a survey at a light-engineering factory employing 3,500 women and also in the branches of a multiple store employing 10,000 women. It showed that 45% of the 269 women reporting sick were in their paramenstruum. Dr. William Bickers and Maribelle Woods from the Medical College of Virginia, as long ago as 1951, noted that 36% of women in their premenstrual week requested sedation during working hours.

A survey in four London hospitals showed that half of all emergency admissions of women to hospitals occurred during the premenstruum. This figure was the same for the medical emergencies, like coronaries and strokes, for the surgical admissions like colic and appendicitis, for infectious fevers and for admissions to the psychiatric wards. Admissions for depression and suicides have been shown the world over to be the highest during the paramenstruum.

Accidents at work are another problem to industry, both the minor cuts and bruises, which are a waste of working time and are treated at the sick bay, and the serious ones admitted to hospital. Research at the U.S. Center for Safety Education showed that the 48 hours before the onset of menstruation are the most dangerous ones when most accidents at work occur. In Germany it was noted that apprentice tightrope walkers had most accidents in the premenstruum. In restaurants it is recognized that the premenstrual clumsiness of waitresses accounts for an undue number of breakages.

The lowering of mental ability during the paramenstruum accounts for unnecessary typing errors and more than one secretary has been referred for treatment when her boss could no longer put up with those few days in each month when letters had to be returned for retyping. Journalists, artists and authors find this a problem too, lacking inspiration and waiting hopefully for a brainwave, which is more likely to come during the postmenstruum. Errors of billing, accounts, stocktaking and filing take longer to correct than to perform, and again the incidence of mistakes is highest during the paramenstruum. Premenstrual irritability may show itself in bad-tempered service by salespeople, receptionists and waitresses, who are in the public eye. Lowered judgment during the premenstruum must also be considered by teachers, magistrates and examiners. Hasty and wrong decisions are the problems of the executives. One teacher wrote with honesty "Every month there are one or two days when I am simply not worth the salary my employers pay me."

There are some specialized occupations which would appear to have their own particular hazards on those premenstrual days, such as the hoarseness which affects opera and other professional singers. One musical comedy star in the 1930s would, with devastating regularity, come into the theater once a month surrounded by a powerful aroma of garlic which preceded her wherever she went. "You see," she would explain, "It's this sore throat again and garlic is the only thing that saves my voice." Sure enough, four days later she would once again be in magnificent voice, but whether it was the garlic or her postmenstruum that was responsible is a matter for guesswork. For artists in the theater the premenstrual syndrome is a very real problem. One great impresario/producer would always attend rehearsal wearing a top hat and smoking a cigar. On one occasion his leading lady was making a fuss and obviously in her premenstruum. The great man stood up in the center of the auditorium, ground his cigar to dust under his feet and hurling his hat on the floor stamped on it crying out "Woman! I don't know why I employ you, you drive me to distraction!" There was a pause and in a changed voice he went on "But when you are well – you're magnificent!"

One wonders how many of the so called "prima donnas"

with their reputation for throwing tantrums were really only reacting to their premenstrual syndrome? For the members of the chorus, the showgirls and ballet dancers, it is always a question of whether the stage manager has enough experience to realize their problem and help them over those difficult days. Their problems of bloatedness and puffy eyes and skin are also shared by models and filmstars who often have a clause in their contracts forbidding filming during the paramenstruum. The lowered sensitivity to taste is a handicap to cooks, who may overflavor the sauces and other foods. Nor must we forget the woman astronaut, Russia's Valentina Tereshkova, who in 1973 had to be brought down after only three days in space when she began to menstruate heavily in the zero gravity.

In Argentina women are allowed under the Constitution to take the necessary days off for their menstrual miseries, and in India wives have long had the privilege of being excused from housework as it is known that any food they prepare may be spoilt.

The site of an individual's premenstrual symptoms may be determined by her work. An investigation into the incidence of the premenstrual syndrome was carried out in a light-engineering factory. About twenty women are interviewed in batches each day. Some days it was noted that the predominant symptom was premenstrual backache, and on other days headache was the commonest symptom. Later it transpired that all the women in any one batch came from the same department and were doing the same kind of work. Those who spent their working hours bending over a workbench were more likely to complain of backache, while those employed sitting at a bench assembling minute electrical parts, a task needing considerable mental concentration, were mostly those complaining of premenstrual headaches.

Texas Instruments found that women had less menstrual absenteeism when they worked from 2:00 P.M. to 10:00 P.M.

compared with the other shifts of 6:00 A.M. to 2:00 P.M. and 8:30 A.M. to 5:30 P.M. Maybe this was because the woman who woke up feeling ill had more time to dose herself and recover from her problems. It is certainly a point worth considering by those who are given an option for choosing their own working hours. Sufferers of the premenstrual syndrome usually cope especially badly with night-shift work, which seems to be because the 'Diurnal Clock,' which determines the hours of sleep and wakefulness, is situated in the hypothalamus and easily disturbs the menstrual clock. This has been found to be a problem with nurses, especially those in training whose regulations demand a specified period of night work. Night work too often leads to upsets of the menstrual pattern and to depressive illnesses in sufferers of the premenstrual syndrome.

The premenstrual syndrome can affect the chances of getting employment, holding the job down, receiving promotion and losing it unnecessarily.

The problems of some sufferers are shown in the following quotations from letters:

"I cannot plan to go anywhere during these depressing times and I live in constant fear of losing my job as I have to take time off each month with a real sick headache. My chances of promotion have been ruined because of this."

"I have recently given up my job unnecessarily and realized that it is ridiculous to let this condition ruin my whole life. Although I know the cause of my depressive feelings I seem to be unable to think logically and though I know I shall be fine again in a week's time I seem to get quite illogical and irrational at the same time."

"I am thirty-three years of age and have suffered from the premenstrual syndrome for the best part of my adult life. The symptoms are horrible depression, muddle-headedness and feeling dead from the neck up. I recently took the totally unnecessary and very impulsive step of resigning from my post as a teacher of English. Of course it was just before my period that I took this drastic step. I am well qualified and have been doing this now for seven years. To all other people I appear cheerful, calm and efficient, especially when a period is not on its way."

A specialized problem has recently arisen in the Ortho Pharmaceuticals oral contraceptive plant in Puerto Rico where breast enlargement has been found among the men and menstrual disorders among the women. This has occurred in spite of the strict precautions taken in making the synthetic estrogens. These include hermetically sealed machines, air conditioning, respirators, and special protective clothing (even down to the underwear). The long-term effects of occupational exposure to estrogens are practically unknown and there are no safety standards in force anywhere.

How can industry cope with this unnecessary financial burden caused by menstrual problems? Fortunately most employers are supplying convenient rest rooms where a woman can relax for a few hours, take something to ease her sufferings and return to continue work for the rest of the day. The availability of flexitime, by which each worker clocks herself in and out of work at times that suit her best, is a boon to many women. They can hold a few hours in hand so that when they are at their lowest they need not go to work for that day.

Perhaps industry should tackle the problem more seriously by educating its staff, especially personnel managers and forewomen, to recognize and fully understand the problems so that women can be assigned to less skilled jobs such as packing and stacking during their vulnerable days, rather than remaining on tasks which are harder to remedy later, such as soldering or filing.

Finally, treatment centers should be available, as these problems are not insoluble and can be treated. Such centers should be available either in hospitals or at centers of employment.

12

Lady's Leisure

Even when she's off duty, away from office and housework and just relaxing, the black cloud of once a month may still be with her. For among those who have led a quiet sedentary life all the week looking forward to the weekend's pleasure on the yacht, up in the mountains, on the cycle or down in the caves, which woman wants to be bothered with menstrual problems? Fortunately there's an answer for those women who are on the pill. They can be asked, when they start their initial course, "Which day of the week would it be most convenient for you to menstruate?" and as menstruation can be expected to occur within two days of stopping the course it does not entail a very difficult calculation to decide on which day to begin. Admittedly there are some who would find it more convenient to menstruate at the weekends, when the husband can take over the tasks and care for the children.

SPORTS

What about the other sporting activities in which women indulge? Those who enjoy a game of club tennis, golf or squash may well find that during the paramenstruum their performance deteriorates, for it has been found that this is the time when the arm and hand steadiness is impaired, the sharpness of vision deteriorates and there may be a slowing of movement with the extra weight and water retention. The menstrual influence on many of our top sportswomen is different, because they are chosen from those women who maintain a steady standard without fluctuations in performance. However, research by the British Women's Amateur Athletics Association confirmed that one group of sportswomen, the top athletes, gave their best performance during their postmenstruum, and in preparation for the 1976 Olympics they arranged menstrual engineering (adjusting the time of menstruation) so that the British athletes at least did not have to rely on Nature's roulette.

Dr. Ken Dyer of Adelaide has produced some interesting figures showing that over the past twenty years women's top athletic performances have improved more than men's, and suggesting that possibly within the next three or four decades women will be running and swimming as well as men, certainly in the longer distance races. Women have determination and aggression and are especially suited to prolonged exertion; they have the striking example of the Canadian, Cynthia Nicolas, who in the summer of 1977 set a new world record for a double crossing of the English Channel in 19 hours 55 minutes, compared with the previous male record of 30 hours.

HOBBIES

Women have so many hobbies that it is difficult to cover them all. There are those women who enjoy dressmaking, but will avoid cutting out a dress in an expensive material on the wrong day of the month for fear of spoiling it. Others will hesitate to spend money on flowers at that time as they find they cannot arrange them to perfection. Artists may well have difficulties and feel their inspiration is lost, and will wait until their postmenstrual peak.

Intellectual games may be affected once a month, as the partner at bridge may have discovered or the opponent at chess or scrabble may well appreciate.

DRIVING HAZARDS

Driving is a leisure time activity of many women; for some it means an active participation in car rallies while for most it is the social journey or outing. In either case there will be a menstrual handicap. A survey at four hospitals showed that half of all accident admissions of women occurred during those vital paramenstrual days. Indeed among those involved in an accident the menstrual influence was equally present among the passengers, passive participants, as among the drivers, active participants. In those few seconds which elapse between the car climbing the curb and before it hits a brick wall the alert passenger may brace herself up and cover her head for protection, while the passenger in her paramenstruum may be too slow or dull to take even these elementary precautions.

Driving is a complicated task requiring the coordination of many skills, which are lowered during the paramenstruum. Complicated and rapidly changing road situations demand instant reaction and good judgment, and if this is lowered there may be an increase in the braking distance. The alertness of hearing is decreased so that the driver may not hear the warning horn. The impaired sharpness of vision and lowered ability to judge shapes and sizes means that she loses her normal precision in parking and reversing the car. She may be impatient of the slow driver ahead or an elderly person crossing the road in front of her car. She may overtake irrationally on a blind bend or drive aggressively round a dangerous corner. She may fail to notice the changing weather conditions, failing light or alterations on the road surfaces. She may forget to fasten her safety belt or to remember the Driving Code. Even as a pedestrian she is still vulnerable in her paramenstruum and may cross the road without the usual precautions, while as a mother she may not be alert enough to stop her child from dangers on the road. Having said all that, perhaps one should add that women are considered by the insurance companies better risks than men; women are at risk only during the paramenstruum, certainly not during the postmenstrual peak.

SHOPPING

The joys of a shopping spree may be marred during the paramenstruum. She may become an indecisive, dithering shopper who tries on all the shoes in the shop, finds they won't fit because of her swollen feet and leaves the shop empty handed. She may buy some totally unwanted dresses, which don't fit and are the wrong color, which she'll never wear. It is possible that her color sense and appreciation of shape and size deteriorate during this phase of the cycle. A few women even buy unnecessary and expensive items, like furs and jewelry, merely to spite the husband. One can't help feeling sorry for the man who wrote:

> "I know it's the wrong day for my wife if I come home and find the kitchen loaded with fruit, anything up to ten pounds of apples, bananas and oranges. I know she'll be in a foul temper and ask me to put the children to bed. But at other times she's the best wife in the world."

There is the problem of women shoplifters, who are caught during the paramenstruum. While it is possible that they really are in a totally confused state and unaware of their action, it is also possible that they are habitual shop-

lifters, who were caught at a time when they were not suffi-
ciently alert and did not take the usual precautions before
indulging in the habit.

ENTERTAINMENTS

Social entertainments may not be all that successful during
the paramenstruum. Cocktail parties too often require prolonged standing which isn't fun for those with water retention. As one woman put it:

> "I can always recognize fellow sufferers as they also edge
> their way towards the walls to rest their legs."

Other problems related to this time of the month are
described:

> "My problem is about ten days before a period comes. I
> get uncontrollable fits of depression which makes me hit
> rock bottom. If I am with a crowd of friends I feel like
> I'm going to suffocate, it's a feeling that comes over me
> and I want to run out, and I do run out."

> "I often have to entertain for my husband. I am a good
> cook even if I say it myself. An excellent meal is ready
> but when the first guest arrives I just burst into tears.
> It ruins my whole evening. I've learnt to arrange my
> dates after my period, but then my period is bound to
> be late!"

Nor can the theater bring pleasure to everyone, as one
sufferer from premenstrual depression recalled:

> "I remember sitting in the theater with tears rolling

down my cheeks – squeezing my hands and saying to myself 'NO – I mustn't, this is a comedy – everyone else is laughing.' "

The problems of alcoholic intoxication are increased during the paramenstruum, so that the woman can never really let herself go without ending up in trouble. Some women can never take cannabis without suffering its worst effects, however there are those women who can take it at most times of the month and enjoy the experience, but if they take it during the paramenstruum they develop delusions or hallucinations.

Some women have an uncontrollable urge to gamble during the premenstruum, and the compulsion is just as bad whether it is on the horses, the dogs or in the bingo hall. One of my patient's addictions is gambling on slot machines; on some days of the month she's just spellbound by them and can't stop. Realizing the habit, she tries to go out without any money to help remove the temptation.

13

The Hormonal Control

Some scientists believe that the body is governed by bio-rhythms, which include a physical rhythm of 23 days, a sensitivity or emotional rhythm of 28 days and an intellectual rhythm of 33 days. These body cycles are not affected by life's events and repeat themselves so unchangingly that they can be worked out for any individual by anyone who can count, or by computer, provided only that the hour and date of birth is known. Under no circumstances should the menstrual cycle be associated with biorhythms, for it is completely different. No matter how precisely you can pin-point the hour and date of birth, this will not enable you or anyone else to work out when the menstrual cycle will begin, what its length will be or anything at all about its pattern of ovulation and menstruation.

The menstrual cycle does not begin at birth. It is inter-rupted by pregnancy and breast feeding, and is altered by life's events such as illnesses, examinations, bereavement, happy events, sad events and changes in environment. Fur-thermore, menstrual patterns show endless variations in duration of flow and quantity of blood lost, as well as in the length of cycle.

When teaching about the menstrual cycle it is easiest if one considers only a 28-day cycle. It makes for simplicity and is easier when discussing the various changes, such as ovulation on the fourteenth day. But we must not lose sight of the fact that women are all individuals and do not fit naturally into such neat pigeon-holes. Sometimes one is asked "What is the right length of the menstrual cycle?" One might as well ask "What is the right height for a woman?" All individuals are different, one meets many healthy normal women who menstruate about every 21 days, as well as those at the other extreme who only menstruate on average every 36 days. Both are quite normal with fully effective reproductive systems. The cycle of 28 days is only the average of all women all over the world.

It is said that Dr. Pinkus, the father of the pill, decided over a cup of tea with the British endocrinologist, Peter Bishop, that 28 days would be a convenient time interval to allow withdrawal bleeding to occur in women on the pill. So it is that today there are millions of women with man-made cycles of 28 days. But they could just as easily have decided on 24 days or 30 days.

Chiazze and his colleagues found that only 62% of women aged 15–19 years had a menstrual cycle between 25 and 31 days, but the proportion of women gradually increased with age so that between 35 and 39 years there were 86% with an almost conventional cycle. When women are asked the length of their cycle the frequent reply is "Oh I'm always late," meaning it is more than 28 days, or "I'm quite regular" meaning "I never have to get worried because I'm never over 28 days." Incidentally, the days of a cycle should always be counted from the first day of menstruation until the first day of the next menstruation. Confusion sometimes occurs because women count from the end of one period until the beginning of the next: they count only the days they are not bleeding.

The duration in the time of menstrual flow varies too from cycle to cycle and from individual to individual. It may be for as short as two days or go on as long as eight days, and still the doctors would consider it normal and know that these women would be able to have children if this was their desire. The quantity of the menstrual flow, or blood loss, is also variable, and as no two people are likely to see another person's flow there is bound to be considerable exaggeration in both directions. Some women will even say "I had a really good period" which can be interpreted as meaning the loss was bright red. Many women object to the scanty dark red, brown or black loss which sometimes comes with the pill. It is as well to realize that menstrual bleeding comes from the minute blood vessels on the lining of the womb, and not from any big blood vessels, so that if bleeding continued for a very long time it might cause anemia, but one can never actually bleed to death as one could from a wound in the limb.

THE MENSTRUAL CONTROLLING CENTER

In the opening chapter the menstrual cycle was broken down into seven four-day phases of hormone activity. Each hormone change is carefully monitored by the control center, often referred to as the "menstrual clock," which is not situated in the womb where the action takes place but at a distance from it, low in the brain, in a part known as the "hypothalamus" where it can receive impulses from the brain. (Figure 17) The hypothalamus is itself the control center of many other functions, among them being the centers for the control of water balance, of appetite, of weight and of mood, so that if any one of these is upset it will tend to affect the others. The diagram in Figure 18 shows the proximity of these centers, which explains why, when the menstrual cycle is disturbed, such as by taking the pill, it can upset the weight, the water balance and the

mood center, causing in turn a gain in weight, water retention and depression. In a similar way, if the appetite is
drastically curtailed, as in anorexia nervosa, the menstrual
cycle will be stopped and depression will develop. Again,
depressive illnesses are likely to cause an alteration in menstruation resulting in either excessive bleeding, as in the
"weeping womb," or stopping menstruation. It can also cause
alterations in weight, either a gain or a loss.

The diurnal controlling center, which is concerned with
sleep rhythms, is also situated in the hypothalamus close to
the menstrual clock. Those with a sensitive menstrual clock
are likely to be easily upset by night shift working, and have
marked jet lag after long flights.

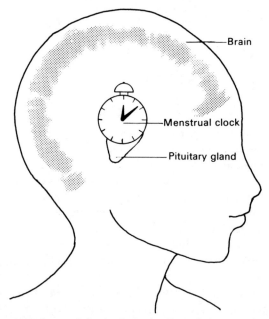

It is at the base of the brain in the Hypothalamus, above
the Pituitary gland.

Figure 17   Position of the menstrual clock

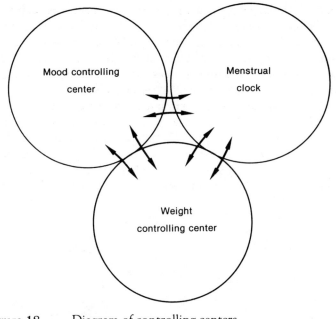

Figure 18   Diagram of controlling centers
in the hypothalamus

MENSTRUAL CLOCK

The Menstrual Clock, being the control center of the menstrual cycle, is responsible for the smooth and effective operation of the woman's marvelous reproductive system. Situated in the hypothalamus, it has two hormones which it uses for this purpose. Hormones are chemicals with their own individual structure and designed to act on a particular target organ. They are chemical messengers traveling in the blood stream. These two hormones have very grand sounding names, "follicle stimulating hormone releasing hormone" (FSHRH) and "luteinising hormone releasing hormone" (LHRH). Their target is the pituitary gland situated next to the hypothalamus at the base of the brain. The effect of these two releasing hormones from the hypothalamus is to stimulate the pituitary gland to produce two other menstrual hormones, follicle stimulating hormone (FSH) and luteinising hormone (LH), boosting the hormone output. (Figure 19)

The pituitary gland sends out a variety of different hormones which control, among other things, growth, pigmentation, lactation, thyroid, adrenal and insulin output. In short it has a finger in every pie. But what concerns us now are the two pituitary hormones, follicle stimulating hormone and luteinising hormone, which act on the ovary. The follicle

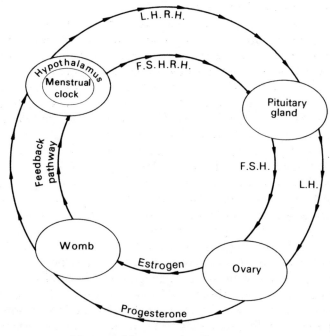

Figure 19   Menstrual hormonal pathways

stimulating hormone acts on the ovaries by stimulating the formation of follicles, or tiny microscopic rings of cells within which is an immature ovum, or egg cell. As the follicles develop, specialized cells produce *estrogen*, yet another hormone, which is released into the blood stream. Estrogen builds up the lining of the womb to replace that which was shed at the last menstruation. But estrogen has another important function. Before ovulation it thins the cervical mucus, or natural vaginal discharge, to assist the sperms entering the womb in their search for the egg cell, which needs to be fertilized before pregnancy can occur. At puberty estrogen is responsible for the development of the secondary sex characteristics, such as breast development, hair growth and the rounded female contours.

At mid-cycle it is the sudden surge of the other pituitary hormone, luteinising hormone, which causes the ripened follicle to burst and discharge its egg cell, a process known as '*ovulation.*' Further stimulation by the luteinising hormone causes new cells to form at the site of the burst follicle, and these cells produce the other menstrual hormone, *progesterone*. Progesterone is secreted in spurts and after ovulation it passes in the blood stream to its target organ, which is the womb. Figure 1 gave the levels of these hormones during a normal menstrual cycle.

After the lining of the womb has been rebuilt under the influence of estrogen it is converted by progesterone into a soft, spongy lining, hopefully ready for the embedding of a fertilized egg. Thus progesterone is only needed after ovulation, when the initial repair work on the lining of the womb has already taken place. Progesterone is also responsible for making the fallopian tubes contract more forcefully but less frequently, so that the egg cell may be swept along to the womb. Progesterone also changes the vaginal discharge from the thin watery fluid, in which sperm could move freely, into a thick sticky mucus, thus preventing further sperm entering the womb. The presence of progesterone raises the body temperature again in preparation for a possible pregnancy.

Nature has devised a magnificent machine in our reproductive system, complete with a highly efficient intercommunication system between the hypothalamus, pituitary, ovary and womb which is called the "feedback pathway." This ensures that the higher centers are kept fully informed of the progress down below (Figure 19) and can alter the level of hormones according to the information received. For instance should conception occur the hormonal output is altered within hours. Another important control is *prolactin*, a hormone produced by the anterior pituitary gland which regulates the progesterone feedback mechanism so that if too much prolactin is produced the progesterone feedback pathway is interrupted.

OVULATION

Most women recognize when ovulation occurs as there may be a slight sensation of discomfort for about an hour in one side of the lower abdomen, and at the same time they may notice that their normal vaginal discharge changes from a thin fluid to a thick, sticky mucus. Some women have a migraine at that time or a tendency to irritability, while for the more unfortunate women it may herald the onset of the premenstrual syndrome. Sometimes when the migraine or irritability at ovulation is severe women have difficulty in becoming pregnant because they avoid having intercourse on the very days that they are most likely to conceive.

If a woman carefully records her temperature for two minutes every morning before getting out of bed it is possible to decide whether or not she is ovulating and also whether she has sufficient progesterone. In Figure 20 a few

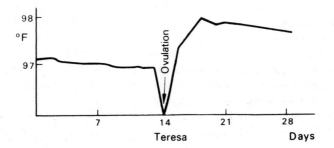

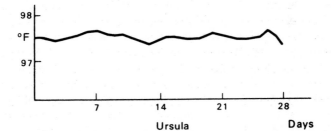

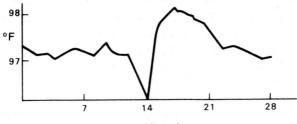

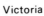

Figure 20   Temperature charts taken through the menstrual cycle

temperature charts are shown. *Teresa* is normal; ovulation occurred as shown by the sudden dip and subsequent raised temperature until the start of menstruation. *Ursula's* chart is very steady, and all on the same level with no evidence of ovulation; it is known as an 'anovular chart.' *Victoria's* chart does show ovulation and a rise of temperature, but this rise is not maintained, suggesting that she has insufficient progesterone.

The exact time of ovulation can be determined in several ways: by the change from a thin discharge to thick sticky mucus, a daily temperature chart, tests showing the time of the peak of luteinising hormone in the blood, and direct inspection of the ovary either at the time of an abdominal operation or by laparascopy, in which a minute periscope is inserted through the abdominal wall. Ovulation occurs 12–14 days before the onset of menstruation, so that it is correct to talk about ovulation at mid-cycle in one whose cycle averages 28 days, but in those who have a longer cycle ovulation will be occurring after mid-cycle as shown in Figure 21. In women with a 35-day cycle ovulation is likely to occur about day 21, whereas in those with a short cycle of 21 days it is more likely to occur about day 10.

EMOTIONAL UPSET
OF MENSTRUATION

The menstrual clock is a very delicate mechanism which requires an exact hormone balance to ensure a trouble free menstruation. It is easily upset by stresses of all kinds, both the happy events such as weddings, holidays and promotion, and the unpleasant stresses like examinations, bereavements, financial and marital problems.

The extent to which emotion can affect the timing of menstruation was shown in a study of 91 boarding school girls, who were all taking their tenth grade high school examinations in the second week of June. The average number of girls menstruating each day before the examinations was sixteen girls, but during the vital examination week as many as thirty-six girls were menstruating on one day. In fact just under half showed an alteration in their normal menstrual pattern. In many the cycle was lengthened, in others it was shortened, in some menstruation lasted longer so that it spread over during examination week but there were about a dozen of those girls who missed menstruation entirely that month. Clinical observation suggests that each individual's reaction to stress has a tendency to be the same throughout their menstruating years, so that the girls who missed menstruation at the time of examinations might also stop suddenly in later life if they were molested or their homes burnt down. The others, who reacted with prolonged menstrual loss, might similarly expect to react in the same way under severe stress.

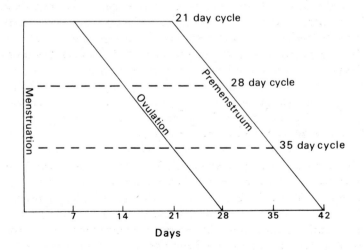

Figure 21   Timing of ovulation with different
                   lengths of cycles

One letter writer asked:

"Since my husband was killed in a sailing accident last year my periods have been very irregular and much heavier. I have now got over the loss, have got a new job and only get depressed before a period. Is this anything to worry about?"

No, a horrible shock like that is bound to be felt by the hypothalamus, which in turn will temporarily upset the normal menstrual pattern. As she appears to be adjusting her life to the tragedy it is likely that gradually her menstruation will return to its old pattern.

MENSTRUAL SYNCHRONY

Another point to be considered in relation to the timing of menstruation is what is called "menstrual synchrony," which is when a number of women's menstruations occur together. This happens among women who live closely together in closed communities like communes, prisons, convents, college campuses and school dormitories, and especially if they share common emotional experiences, such as examinations and end of term excitement, their menstruation gradually becomes synchronized. This in turn raises fresh problems for it also means that if more than one woman is suffering from premenstrual tension trouble is inevitable. Indeed it may be necessary to move women prisoners from one cell to another before such synchronization occurs. Menstrual synchrony is frequently noticed with mothers and daughters. If a daughter is brought to the doctor by her mother and is unable to remember the date of her last menstruation, the chances are that the mother will reply and then add "our dates always come together." Similarly menstruation tends to coincide in lesbians. The mechanism of this synchronization is not clear, but it has been suggested that it may be related to sensitive body odors.

The potency of these menstrual hormones is almost unbelievable. The powder a woman uses to cover the tip of her nose weighs many times more than the total amount of female hormones to be found in her blood stream. Yet they cause the sex organs and breasts to grow to mature size, and they bring about changes in bone structure and fat distribution which mould her figure into feminine contours and bring her to the peak of womanhood and motherhood.

14

What Goes Wrong?

THE PREMENSTRUAL SYNDROME

There are many factors which suggest that progesterone deficiency is the cause of the premenstrual syndrome. For instance:

1) The symptoms are only present when progesterone should be present in the blood stream, i.e. after ovulation up to menstruation. (Figure 22) The symptoms disappear when progesterone is absent from the bloodstream i.e. after menstruation.

2) The onset is usually either at puberty, after a pregnancy, after pill-taking, or when menstruation returns after a long absence: all times of hormonal upset.

3) There is a frequent absence of symptoms during pregnancy when high amounts of progesterone are produced by the placenta.

4) Temperature charts confirm that the rise after ovulation is poorly sustained in sufferers of the premenstrual syndrome. (See Victoria's temperature chart, Figure 20.)

5) The average progesterone level after ovulation is lower in sufferers of the premenstrual syndrome than in normal women without menstrual symptoms. (Figure 23) Professor R. Taylor of the Premenstrual Clinic at St. Thomas's Hospital, London, found that

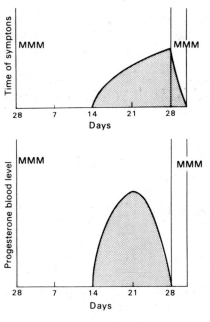

Figure 22   Time of premenstrual syndromes and progesterone level during the menstrual cycle

out of 105 patients with the premenstrual syndrome roughly half had a lowered progesterone level in the second half of the cycle.

Recently the biochemists have developed a new technique known as "radioimmunoassay" by which it is possible to measure a minute quantity of a biological substance, such as progesterone, in the blood. This has been a great advance but it is still a difficult and expensive technique, only available for research purposes at present. It must be remembered that progesterone is produced in spurts into the blood stream, which makes the interpretation of results difficult.

Merely to say that there is a progesterone deficiency still leaves many questions waiting for an answer. For example:

a) Is there insufficient production of progesterone from the ovary?

b) Is there insufficient luteinising hormone (LH) produced by the pituitary gland?

c) Is there insufficient luteinising hormone releasing hormone (LHRH) produced by the hypothalamus?

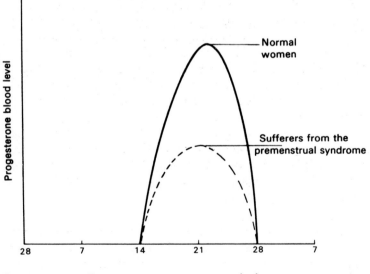

Figure 23   Progesterone in patients with the premenstrual syndrome and in normal women

d) Is the progesterone deficiency a true deficiency or merely in comparison to the high estrogen so often found in sufferers of the syndrome?

e) Is the progesterone feedback pathway being blocked by too high a level of prolactin produced by the pituitary gland?

It is probable that cases of the premenstrual syndrome fall into one or more of these groups, but up to now we have not been able to differentiate these factors. Recently my daughter, Maureen Dalton M.D., has developed a blood test of value in diagnosing premenstrual syndrome and differentiating it from menstrual distress. It estimates the binding capacity of Sex Hormone Binding Globulin (SHBG). As reported in the Post Graduate Hospital Journal in September 1981, the SHBG levels were estimated in fifty women with severe and well-diagnosed premenstrual syndrome, and in each case the result was below the expected level of 50–80 DHT binding capacity. It is a valuable test, but cannot be performed if the woman is taking any type of medication or if she is unduly hairy. Furthermore the low SHBG level in premenstrual syndrome patients rises when they are given progesterone, the rise being higher when higher doses of progesterone are given.

THE TIME OF ONSET

The onset of the premenstrual syndrome is either at puberty, after a pregnancy or the pill. In those cases which start at puberty the progesterone deficiency will have been present since the start of menstruation. During pregnancy considerably higher levels of progesterone are continuously present in the blood for nine months, and not just present for two weeks and then absent for two weeks as in the non-pregnant woman. During the early weeks of pregnancy this extra pro-

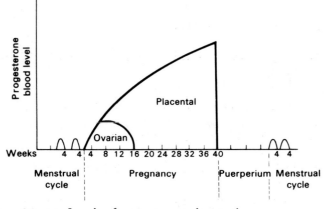

Figure 24   Levels of progesterone during the
menstrual cycle and pregnancy

gesterone is produced by the ovary, and as the placenta, or
afterbirth, develops in the womb it becomes a progesterone
factory producing greater and greater amounts of progesterone. (Figure 24) During labor, after the baby is born, the
placenta, or progesterone factory, comes away and some
women find difficulty in adjusting again to producing sufficient ovarian progesterone and it is these who develop the
premenstrual syndrome. They are often women whose pregnancies have been complicated by pre-eclampsia (high blood
pressure and swelling of the ankles) or postnatal depression.

The pill contains a man-made artificial steroid called a
'*progestogen*' which acts as a contraceptive and which also
lowers the progesterone level in the blood (Figure 31, p. 186).
This means the pill produces a progesterone deficiency in
those women whose progesterone production is not flexible
enough to counteract the action of the progestogen.

The symptoms of the premenstrual syndrome are many
and various, but they all come under one or more of the
following headings:

1) Water retention.

2) Lowered blood sugar.

3) Excess sodium and insufficient potassium at cellular level.

4) Allergic reactions, e.g. asthma, rhinitis.

5) Lowered resistance to infection, e.g. boils, styes.

6) Inflammatory reactions, e.g. conjunctivitis.

It is possible that the symptoms related to water retention, lowered blood sugar and altered sodium and potassium levels are due to a disturbance of the respective controlling centers in the hypothalamus. This is also a possible explanation for the last three, alternatively there may be an upset in the adrenal gland, for progesterone is also produced in the adrenals where it is converted into the various adrenal hormones, or corticosteroids. The corticosteroids have many functions, including that of mobilizing the mechanisms responsible for fighting infections and dealing with allergic reactions and inflammation.

From all this it follows that the specific treatment of the premenstrual syndrome is to make good the deficiency by administering progesterone. Information on progesterone treatment is given in Chapter 18.

FALL IN BLOOD SUGAR LEVEL

Some attacks of the premenstrual syndrome are triggered off by fasting, causing a fall in blood sugar level. This is often the cause of sudden aggressive outbursts, migraine, panics and epilepsy. Figure 25 shows a simplified figure of blood sugar levels and the effect of taking food. If the blood sugar level is too high the patient is a diabetic, but we will only consider here what happens in normal healthy women whose blood sugar level remains within the normal limits. When a woman takes some food, such as a breakfast of egg and toast, the blood sugar level rises immediately and then falls gradually over the next four hours. If she takes some more food after three or four hours the blood sugar will again rise immediately and then fall slowly. However, if she does not take any food for a long interval the blood sugar will continue to drop until it reaches the baseline. In a normal healthy woman the blood sugar will not be able to fall below this baseline because of one of those ingenious fail-safe controls which Nature has provided. Instead, when the blood sugar touches the baseline there is a sudden outpouring of adrenalin which mobilizes some of the sugar stored in the body, and the blood sugar rises again. However, when the

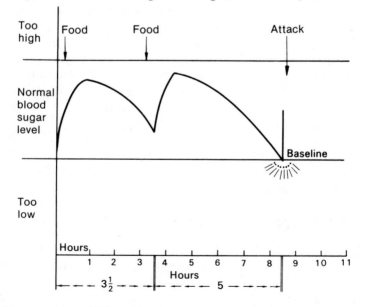

Figure 25   Effect of food on blood sugar levels

sugar is taken from the cells they fill up with water and this is responsible for water retention, bloatedness and weight gain.

Adrenalin is the hormone which also mobilizes the body's defences against "fright, fight and flight," and this sudden outpouring of adrenalin may be enough to trigger off a sudden fit of irritability, migraine, panic or epilepsy. In others it may cause them to feel weak, shivery, faint or bring on palpitations. On the other hand there are also those fortunate individuals who can manage long fasts, as they are unaware when their blood sugar baseline has been reached and they get renewed energy from their own sugar stores.

These attacks brought on by fasting are sometimes erroneously called "hypoglycemic attacks," but doctors don't like that word as "hypoglycemia" is reserved for those whose blood sugar stays below the baseline and below the normal

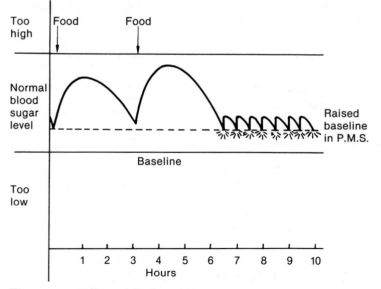

Figure 26 Effect of food on blood sugar levels in sufferers from premenstrual syndrome

blood sugar level. In the case of normal women Nature's fail-safe control prevents hypoglycemia occurring.

The reason why these fasting attacks are often worse before and during menstruation is because at this time the change in hormone levels alters the sugar tolerance and raises the level of the lower baseline, so that the blood sugar level does not have so far to drop before the surge of adrenalin occurs. Many women will have noticed that they can easily diet and go five hours without food after menstruation, but they have marked food cravings before menstruation. Giving progesterone helps to correct this premenstrual alteration of the blood sugar level.

SPASMODIC DYSMENORRHEA

It has already been mentioned that spasmodic dysmenorrhea is the opposite to the premenstrual syndrome and there are several factors which suggest that estrogen deficiency lies at the cause of these period pains. For instance:

1) It does not start with the first menstruation, but only when ovulation occurs.

2) It is relieved by a full-term pregnancy.

3) If a pregnancy does not intervene, a gradual reduction in pain after the age of 25 years is usual.

4) The pain is relieved by the pill or estrogen administration.

5) The sufferers tend to be immature, with poor breast development and sparse hair in their armpits.

6) It is frequently accompanied by acne.

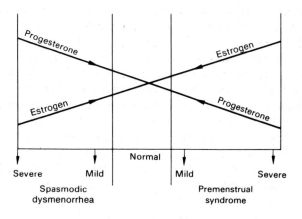

Figure 27   Arbitrary levels of progesterone and estrogen

In puberty, estrogen is responsible for the development of the secondary sex characteristics. It is responsible for the pubertal breast development, for the development of hair in the armpits and lower abdomen, for the development and enlargement of the womb, and more especially for developing the muscles of the womb and ensuring it has a good blood supply. Estrogen decreases the production of grease in the skin and so prevents acne.

If ovular menstruation occurs before the womb is fully developed, the door to the womb is not supple enough to open easily for the flow of menstrual blood. It is rather like trying to blow up a balloon for the first time, which is very difficult, but if it has once been fully inflated then on the next occasion it is easy to inflate. If the womb is gradually stretched during the nine months of pregnancy then subsequently the door will open up at menstruation without pain. Or if the muscles of the womb are gradually increased by the prolonged action of estrogen the painful periods are gradually eased during the mid-twenties.

TWO HORMONAL TYPES

Thus it would seem that the two common period problems, the premenstrual syndrome and spasmodic dysmenorrhea, are related to a deficiency in the levels of the two menstrual hormones progesterone and estrogen respectively. Figure 27 shows a diagram of the effect of these two hormone levels on an individual. A marked progesterone deficiency will cause severe premenstrual syndrome, while a mild deficiency will cause only mild premenstrual syndrome. On the other hand a moderately low estrogen level will only cause mild spasmodic dysmenorrhea, but a severe estrogen deficiency will cause severe period pains. In between these two are those fortunate women who do not experience any problems with menstruation. Although women may move slightly up and down this scale during the course of their life, the movement will tend to stay within the limits of the same group, unless either progesterone or estrogen is given or a pregnancy occurs. These two groups of women tend to have other common characteristics.

PROGESTERONE DEFICIENT GROUP

Women in the premenstrual syndrome group will tend to be fertile, but their pregnancies may be followed by post-natal depression, and they are more prone to depressive illnesses and high blood pressure during their life span. Among those who become pregnant one in every five will be likely to have pre-eclamptic toxemia, with a marked gain in weight and high blood pressure during pregnancy, while the others will blossom in pregnancy, being free from their usual premenstrual migraine, asthma and depression, and will later look back on the last months of pregnancy as the healthiest days of their life. These women, if given estrogen, will tend to get side effects as they already have a high level of this hormone. They will be prone to minor side effects of nausea, gain in weight, headaches and depression, but will also risk the more serious ones like thrombosis. The pill contains estrogen, together with a synthetic progestogen, and as already mentioned progestogens lower the normal progesterone level in the blood, so making their existing progesterone deficiency worse.

ESTROGEN DEFICIENT GROUP

On the other hand, the women with spasmodic dysmenorrhea will grow out of their period pains, either following pregnancy or during the mid-twenties, and thereafter will have trouble-free menstruation. These are the women who feel positively better on the pill, even preferring the ones with the relatively higher dose of estrogen, as these boost their low estrogen levels. However at the menopause their already low estrogen levels are not helped by the declining estrogen output from the ovaries, so these women are likely to develop their menopausal symptoms early, even before menstruation has stopped, and unless they are given estrogen replacement treatment during the menopausal years they are likely to be the ones who suffer most from the ending of their child-bearing years.

As with other hormonal disorders it is not surprising to find that there is a marked family tendency with daughters, sisters and mother belonging to the same menstrual hormonal group, either progesterone deficient or estrogen deficient.

MISSED PERIODS

"Married hopes and unmarried fear
Are the common causes of amenorrhea"

Amenorrhea is the absence of periods, and the above

quoted nurses' jingle is a reminder that the commonest cause of a missed menstruation is pregnancy. Often, if the girl is single, it is more likely to be a delayed period. She normally has a long cycle of perhaps 33–36 days, and because she had not kept a record of her cycles and has run a risk during the month she is fearful, on every day after the 28th day, that she might be pregnant. Unfortunately, as yet, the routine pregnancy test cannot be used reliably until two weeks after the missed period, or 42 days since the last period, and this is an awful long time to wait. There is a new blood test, very expensive and not yet routinely available, which can recognise pregnancy within seven days of conception. Today doctors are warned against using the hormone pregnancy test, (two or three tablets of estrogen and progestogen which causes a withdrawal bleed if there is no pregnancy), because of the danger of fetal abnormality if the woman is pregnant and the pregnancy continues. However, there would usually be the tell-tale signs of an early pregnancy such as morning sickness, getting up to urinate at night and painful enlarging breasts.

Missed periods may occur quite normally at puberty, during the first three years after the onset of menstruation, during breast feeding and again at the menopause. In the last case, menstruation has often started to get shorter and the loss lighter before a period is actually missed.

To find the other causes of missed menstruation one must return to the hormonal controlling system, for any upset to the hormonal pathway may disturb the normal rhythm of menstruation. Stress is perhaps the commonest cause:

A friend *Winifred*, with two children, had been visiting us but when she returned to her home she found a fire engine outside and her house aflame. She stopped mensturating for eleven weeks.

Nor is it necessary for the stress to be so unpleasant; it can just as easily happen following happy circumstances.

Yvonne, a 25-year-old graphic artist, had a wonderful romance on a Greek island and stopped menstruating for nine weeks after she returned.

In both these cases it was the result of messages from the brain affecting the menstrual clock situated in the hypothalamus.

Factors which alter the other controlling centers in the hypothalamus (see Figure 18) will also upset the menstrual clock. Common among these are rapid weight changes, especially anorexia nervosa or even rigid dieting which does not quite reach the proportions of anorexia nervosa. In these cases menstruation will not return until the weight returns near to the level at which menstruation last occurred. Depressive illnesses are also likely to delay menstruation, and again it is unlikely to return naturally until the depression is a thing of the past. Other chronic systemic illnesses, such as tuberculosis and acute rheumatic fever, can halt menstruation temporarily.

Lack of menstruation after stopping the pill is an example where the ovary has been prevented from ovulating for so long that the menstrual clock has also been halted, and even when the pill is no longer being taken the menstrual clock does not restart automatically. Often when it does restart after a long interval, the cycles are found to be anovular. This indicates that ovulation has not restarted although menstruation has, and pregnancy is therefore impossible. Fortunately, nowadays, this can be corrected by appropriate hormone treatment.

TOO MUCH

Another problem is when menstruation goes on for too long, comes too often or is too heavy – in short, there is too much of it. Again stress can be the cause, although never in those women who on other occasions miss their menstruation at times of stress.

> *Zena*, a 45-year-old wife of a T.V. producer, bled for nine weeks continuously, starting on the day her dream house, on which she had already put a deposit, was sold to a higher bidder without her knowledge.

There is an interesting example in Mark's Gospel:

"And there was a woman who had a flow of blood for twelve years, and who had suffered much under many physicians, and had spent all that she had, and was no better, but rather grew worse. She had heard the reports about Jesus, and came up behind him in the crowd and touched his garment. For she said "If I touch even his garments, I shall be made well." And immediately the hemorrhage ceased, and she felt in her body that she was healed of her disease." (5, 25–29, RSV)

This incident can be seen in the light of our present medical knowledge. This woman had faith, and the tremendous emotional stress of being able actually to go up and touch the clothes that Jesus was wearing was sufficient stimulus to her menstrual clock to correct her prolonged menstruation.

Hormone therapy, when taking the pill and more especially the progestogen-only pill, may cause prolonged breakthrough bleeding, which can be a great nuisance and is a sign that treatment needs adjusting.

Occasionally there may be bleeding at ovulation; this is usually lighter and only lasts from an hour or two to one or two days, but if there is no regular record of the bleeding it may not be easily recognized. A menstrual chart will clearly show the difference between the regular mid-cycle bleeding, which is harmless, and the totally irregular bleeding which needs gynecological investigation.

Conditions which increase the surface area of the lining of the womb will result in heavy or prolonged bleeding. Examples are polyps, or fibroids which are situated near the cavity of the womb. However, as there is always the chance that the extra bleeding may be the result of a malignant condition, there is always justification in asking for a full examination.

Occasionally an intra-uterine device, whether a coil, loop or copper seven, may cause excessive bleeding or prolonged scanty bleeding for several days before and after menstruation. Although hormone treatment may be tried to stop the excessive bleeding, it is often best to remove the device and reinsert another in a more comfortable position in the womb. Sometimes a device has been in for years without any trouble, and then gradually menstruation gets more prolonged. This is usually a sign that the device is starting to dislodge and may indeed be pushed out of the womb into the vagina.

Sometimes the bleeding which is thought to be menstrual is due to the bleeding of an ulcer, or erosion, at the cervix or opening of the womb. This can easily be spotted by a doctor on examination and he may well cauterize it.

15

The Vacant Plot

Can anyone blame the woman, who for years has endured wretched miseries each month, if she dreams of the day when those troublesome organs are removed by one clean swoop of the surgeon's knife? Already it is such a commonplace procedure that it is known as the Birthday Operation, to be celebrated during the 40th year. Today the operative risks associated with the removal of the womb are minimal, but is it really an answer to a woman's prayers?

It is no good asking the gynecologist, for he sees the woman a few months later, examines the scar to ensure it's well healed, assures her that she'll never again menstruate, possibly prescribes some estrogen tablets and says goodbye. It is better to ask the family doctor, who cares for this woman, not just for one year, but for the next twenty.

There are many very good reasons for the removal of the womb, and possibly the ovaries as well. At the top of that list would come any possibility of malignancy and no doctor will disagree here. Sometimes it is performed because of fibroids, when they are either so large that they are interfering with some other organ, or so numerous that they are causing heavy menstruation; or because of endometriosis, and again these cases are certainly justified. On the other end of the scale there are those women who demand it so as to be 100% contraceptively safe, probably feeling that they cannot run the very small risk with the pill or a device, or possibly having already tried these methods without success. A 42-year-old owner of a boutique confessed that she changed her gynecologist seven times before she found one prepared to remove her womb merely for contraception. She stated that she was not convinced that sterilization would be reliable enough.

Far too many women have the operation in order to overcome their premenstrual syndrome. They would be better advised to have this condition treated with progesterone therapy. No one will disagree that on many occasions the symptoms are so severe that drastic treatment is warranted, but unfortunately a hysterectomy is not the answer. One well-known gynecologist diagnoses premenstrual syndrome, explains to the woman that this is due to progesterone deficiency, does a hysterectomy and then refers her to the Premenstrual Syndrome Clinic for progesterone treatment.

Many of the problems for which the operation is recommended could alternatively be treated much more successfully with hormone therapy.

The immediate post-operative weeks are usually good and uneventful, but whether the womb only or the womb plus the ovaries are removed, there is still an irreparable break in the hormonal pathway (Figure 19) and the menstrual clock, which is not touched at operation, receives a severe jolt. Within six to eight days there is an increase in follicle stimulating hormone (FSH) from the pituitary and within eight to ten days an increase in luteinising hormone (LH). The menstrual clock is reacting to the lack of information from the womb, and within a further three weeks there is a threefold increase in follicle stimulating hormone and a twofold increase in luteinising hormone. This occurs whether or not the ovaries have been removed, although the increase is not so great if an estrogen implant is given at the time of operation.

The changes which occur with the surgical removal of

the womb or ovaries are known as an "artificial" menopause, and should not be confused with the natural menopause. In a natural menopause, the changes are very gradual over several years, with a slow closing down of the menstrual clock and shrinking of the ovaries and womb, but in an artificial menopause the changes are sudden and only affect the womb and/or the ovaries, leaving the menstrual clock intact.

All goes well after the operation for some 6–12 months, but then the difference between the two hormonal groups of women discussed on page 136 begins to show itself. Those who previously suffered from the premenstrual syndrome will find that the usual cyclical symptoms return. Often it is the husband who is the first to notice it and he will try to remind the wife of what is happening. Or she may recognize the telltale headache, which previously ushered in a period, and now assumes the proportions of a prostrating migraine.

Angela, the 48-year-old wife of a USAF colonel, had a successful hysterectomy for fibroids which were causing heavy bleeding. She made an excellent recovery and assumed full household duties until nine months later, when she suddenly had four days of extreme tiredness. She stayed in bed attributing it to 'flu or some nasty virus. The following month it recurred, but this time she stayed in bed for six days. Gradually the duration of the tiredness lengthened until it represented two weeks in each month. It would start gradually with mere tiredness and she would manage to keep up for a few days, but then bed became essential. The end of the attacks was quite definite, and afterwards she had no other symptoms and resumed her normal social life.

Her husband had kept a meticulous diary, from which a chart was constructed. When first seen she had already had nine months of this distressing condition which fortunately responded completely to progesterone treatment.

Invariably the premenstrual syndrome is more marked after a hysterectomy than before, and there may also be extra symptoms.

One woman, a part-time worker, was first seen after she had been charged at the police station. Two years previously a hysterectomy had been carried out. Prior to the operation she had suffered from premenstrual tension and headaches.

After the operation her premenstrual syndrome had increased in severity and for a few days each month she would also experience breast fullness and a distressing feeling of unreality and confusion. She related these episodes to the time of her expected premenstruum and carefully charted the days on a calendar. She even went so far as to arrange her working days so as to avoid these inevitable confused days. In Court she described these days of confusion, explaining that sometimes she would come home having bought items she did not need, such as dog food when she had no dogs, curry and other foods which she never ate, and underwear which was the wrong size. She was in a daze and could not recall what had happened. The day of her offence had been such a day. Even when she was taken to the police station by a plain-clothes policeman after having been charged, she thought the officer was a rapist driving down an unknown road. The case was dismissed. She has since been under progesterone treatment, and is now free from cyclical confusion and the premenstrual syndrome.

While carrying out a nationwide survey into the hormonal factors in migraine in women in 1975, it was noted that it was those women with a history of the premenstrual syndrome who stated that the severity of their migraine had been increased by the hysterectomy. Their three-month charts, giving the precise timing of migraine attacks, confirmed that the attacks were still occurring cyclically.

One cannot emphasize too strongly the need for women with cyclical symptoms to keep a careful record of their problem days, even if they have had their womb or ovaries removed. Sometimes when women feel very depressed and are unable to record their days of depression because the onset is so gradual, it is just as useful for them to record the days on which they have breast symptoms, as these are usually very definite and commonplace. Alternatively they can just record the days when they are feeling really well with a [✓].

> Brenda, a 47-year-old, began her consultation with a detailed account of how her husband had been moved from one town to another, how she had made a suicidal attempt within days of arriving there and had been hospitalized for several months. Within a week or two of her discharge she moved back to her previous home, but made another suicide attempt the following week and was again admitted. It was only after a long and confused history, assisted by her husband, that mention was made of a hysterectomy and the fact that she was now experiencing cyclical attacks of depression and moodiness. Once the cyclical nature of her symptoms was appreciated and confirmed by a two-month record it was possible to give her progesterone treatment and restore her to normality.

Two recent surveys have emphasized the high incidence of depression occurring in women one to three years after a hysterectomy, with or without the removal of the ovaries. The depression appears to be greatest in those under 40 years at the time of the operation; those with a previous history of depression, especially postnatal depression; those in whom no gynecological abnormality could be found by the pathologist who examined the womb after operation (in one of the surveys 45% of the wombs were reported to be normal), and in those women who had a history of marital disruption.

Dr. Donald Richards, a general practitioner in Oxford, England, realized that those patients who had previously had a hysterectomy were the patients whose medical notes were bulging out of their files, so that at a glance one realized that they had already done the rounds of most hospital departments. His survey, confirmed by others, emphasized the high incidence of depression in those with a history of a hysterectomy.

My paper on "The Aftermath of Hysterectomy" read at the Royal Society of Medicine in London in 1957 revealed that 44% of women had either been divorced, separated or had sought the assistance of a marriage guidance conselor since the operation. When the woman is ill each month with menstrual problems the husband is more sympathetic than he is when, after the operation, she flies into rages for no apparently accountable reason. One husband said "She used to have a reason for it, but now she's quite unpredictable," and another, "I hoped the operation would make her more even tempered."

Another disturbing finding in the survey was that more than half the women gained more than 28 lbs. in the year following their hysterectomy. How often is a woman warned before the operation that the odds are two to one that such a marked weight gain might occur? The reason for the depression and weight gain after hysterectomy may be appreciated by recognising the proximity of the menstrual clock to the mood controlling center and the weight controlling center in the hypothalamus. (Figure 18)

There would seem to be two types of post-hysterectomy depression, a cyclical depression and a continuous depression. The continuous depression is likely to be suffered by those who in their youth experienced spasmodic dysmenorrhea and have a tendency to be estrogen deficient. These women respond perfectly to estrogen therapy, which needs to be continued not only until their depressive illness is past but well after the time of the natural menopause.

In theory the removal of the womb should have no effect on subsequent sexual activity, in fact it should be enhanced once the fear of a possible pregnancy is permanently removed. The vagina and clitoris are untouched at operation. In practice there are those who previously had a satisfactory sex life, and now suddenly find they have lost all urge and satisfaction. During intercourse when the climax is reached, there is a rhythmic dilation of the upper part of the vagina with a constriction of the lower vagina. If the womb has been totally removed the cervix, which forms the top of the vagina, will have been removed, thus altering the shape of the upper part of the vagina, the part so essential to reaching a full orgasm. A few women are found to have a high prolactin level, suggesting that the operation has caused a disturbance in the hypothalamic-pituitary mechanism. These women respond well to bromocriptine, a drug which lowers the prolactin level.

Perhaps it is relevant to mention that when apes have had their wombs removed their partner also rejects them, but if the ape has only been given a mock operation, without the womb being removed, the couple enjoy a natural sexual relationship. Whether a similar effect occurs in humans is not yet known: one can only guess.

16

Menopausal Miseries

It is only children who long to grow old – adults hate the very thought of it. This is never more true than when the menopause approaches, for this may be seen as a door leading to senility, when it is really the gateway to an era of serenity which is characterized by confidence, calmness, sophistication, stable mood and endless energy.

Women are unique in the animal kingdom as the only females who outlive their reproductive function and can enjoy up to half their life span without it. The end of menstruation occurs according to an individual pre-arranged plan. The menstrual clock runs at its own individual rate, in some it runs on a little longer and in others it stops earlier.

Actually, the word "menopause" means the pausing of menstruation, and more precisely, the last menstruation. It is the reverse of the menarche, but it cannot be timed as accurately because it is only seen in retrospect; only when there have been no further menstruations for a year can it be dated exactly. The term "climacteric" was used to cover the years before and after the last menstruation, a time when the changes in the reproductive system were occurring, but nowadays it is usual to use the term "menopause" more loosely to cover those years of hormonal change.

HORMONAL CHANGES

As with all the changes Nature makes in our reproductive system those at the menopause are very gradual, taking 5–7 years to complete. First there is the gradual missing of ovulation. Studies in which small sections of the normal lining of the womb have been removed and examined microscopically have suggested that the occasional anovular cycle can occur up to six years before the last menstruation. Gradually, missed ovulations become more frequent and with it the menstrual flow may become lighter and scanty. As the ovary is declining, the hypothalamus and pituitary try to stimulate it with an increased output of the two hormones, follicle stimulating hormone (FSH) and luteinising hormone (LH). But the ovaries are unable to respond and cannot increase their production of estrogen and progesterone, which gradually decreases until some years later it comes to an end.

It has already been stated that the main function of estrogen is the rebuilding of the lining of the womb after it has been shed at menstruation, the alteration of the cervical mucus to assist fertilization and for breast development. Estrogen also has some other functions, which are of importance after the menstruating years are finished. Estrogen promotes the cholesterol balance, it is involved in the building up of bones, it nourishes the blood circulatory system and it increases the elasticity of the skin. When estrogen is no longer produced by the ovaries, it continues to be produced in the two adrenal glands, which have always produced a small amount, and in the peripheral tissues. After the menopause it is this non-ovarian estrogen which now has to fulfill the other functions to the blood, bones and skin. All too often there is insufficient for these other tasks, either temporarily during the changeover time or permanently, and it is this lack of estrogen which is responsible for all the unpleasant symptoms of the menopause. All too often the woman, once her ovaries decline, is left to carry on with an insufficiency of this vital and powerful female hormone.

Up to the age of 40 years, narrowing of the arteries, and particularly narrowing of the blood vessels of the heart are between ten to forty times more common in men than in women. After the menopause there is a marked increase in this incidence in women as the circulating estrogen decreases, so that gradually the differences between the men and women becomes less, but it is not until the age of 75 years that the incidence is equal. After a hysterectomy the incidence of narrowing of the arteries and of the coronary vessels is increased fourfold compared with premenopausal women. Also, among those few women who have a premature menopause before the age of 40 years there is a sevenfold increase in coronary thrombosis. So the presence of estrogen in the blood is very important in preventing narrowing of the arteries and the occurrence of coronary disease.

Bones are not stable, unchanging structures. All the time during life, new bone cells are being laid down and old ones removed. This needs calcium, phosphorus and other minerals, vitamins and also estrogen. This is why throughout life everyone, men, women and children included, has a small amount of estrogen circulating in the blood. This estrogen is produced by the two adrenal glands. After the menopause some women, who have relied during their menstruating life on the estrogen produced by the ovaries, may find they have insufficient estrogen being made by the adrenals and this leads to thinning of the bones. This thinning of the bones shows up on X-rays, and ten years after the menopause it is present in 40% of all women. Although this can be halted with estrogen administration, it takes another ten years before the X-rays show any improvement.

Progesterone is not required anymore to prepare the

lining of the womb or the cervical mucus for possible pregnancy after menstruation ceases, but progesterone also has another function. All through life, in both sexes, progesterone is also built up in the adrenal glands from cholesterol, and then immediately converted into estrogen, testosterone, cortisone and the other adrenal hormones, or corticosteroids, which have many and various jobs to do throughout the body. However, as ovarian progesterone was only present in the blood stream for half of each cycle, the adrenals generally managed to make sufficient for their own need during the menstruating years, and so they are usually capable of carrying on this task after the menopause. This is why after the menopause progesterone deficiency is no longer a problem.

TWO HORMONAL GROUPS

Earlier the two hormonal types, the estrogen-deficient and progesterone-deficient, were discussed, but apart from spasmodic dysmenorrhea most of the previous chapters have dealt with the progesterone-deficient group and the havoc that can be caused by the premenstrual syndrome in the home, at work and at leisure. At the menopause we again return to the estrogen-deficient group, for these are the women whose menopausal sufferings begin earliest and are the most severe. This can be seen in Figure 28, which shows that those women who had spasmodic dysmenorrhea in their teens and then sufficient estrogen for normal menstruation nevertheless suffer most from menopausal symptoms, indeed the chances are that they will be experiencing menopausal symptoms while their menstruation is still regularly occurring each month. Their need for estrogen therapy at the menopause is essential and they are the ones who will probably need it for many years to come. Those who were in the normal category may require estrogen therapy during

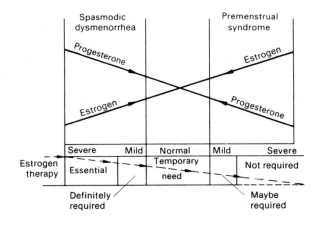

Figure 28   Need for estrogen therapy at the menopause

the changeover period, but they will then probably manage to make sufficient for their own requirements. The sufferers of mild premenstrual syndrome may require estrogen temporarily when their menstruations first stop, but should gradually manage without. On the other hand the severe premenstrual syndrome sufferers are those who will probably have no need for estrogen either during the menopausal years or later; these women have always managed to have a high estrogen level by supplementing the ovarian estrogen with that which is produced in the adrenals.

In short it is a case of roundabouts and swings. Those who had greatest difficulties with monthly problems can look forward to a problem-free era, whilst those who had little trouble during the twenties and thirties are the ones with most problems at the menopause.

It will be noted that the term "Hormone Replacement Treatment" or HRT, has not been used because this only leads to confusion, for both estrogen and progesterone are hormones and both are used in replacement therapy.

AGE OF MENOPAUSE

In the United States the average age of the menopause is 52 years, in Britain it is 48 years, with a range between 45 and 55 years. Those whose menstruation ceases before 45 years are said to have a "premature menopause."

The exact time of the menopause is very individual, however a study of the following four factors can give some indication as to whether it will be early or late:

1) The age of menarche. The effect of this is that those who start menstruation early tend to finish late, giving a "rainbow" effect as shown in Figure 29.

2) The hormonal group. Those in the estrogen-deficient group have a tendency to finish menstruation before the average, while sufferers from the premenstrual syndrome tend to finish after 50 years of age.

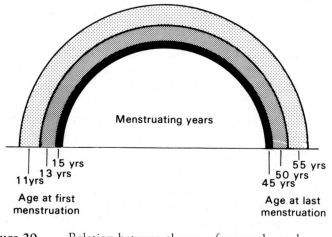

Menstruating years

15 yrs
13 yrs
11yrs

Age at first menstruation

55 yrs
50 yrs
45 yrs

Age at last menstruation

Figure 29   Relation between the age of menarche and menopause

3) Genetic factor. Some families give a story of the mother, sister and aunts all finishing menstruation early, in which case such a patient may also expect to finish early. For this reason it is worth finding out at what age the mother had her last normal menstruation.

4) Smoking. A survey at the BUPA Medical Center in London showed that at 48–49 years 36% of smokers were post-menopausal compared with 23% non-smokers, four years later the figures were 89% smokers and 71% non-smokers. So smoking habits should also be considered when estimating the probable age at which the menopause may occur.

PATTERNS OF ENDING

Among those women who are regularly recording the dates of their menstruation, it can be seen that the menstruating years end in a wide variety of ways. Three patterns are recognized, but even then some women may find that their own individual ending covers more than one pattern:

a) There may be a gradual ending, so that whereas menstruation initially lasted four or five days, it gradually lasts one or two days, then only one day or even one hour monthly, but nevertheless the cycle is maintained and menstruation comes when expected.

b) There may be the occasional missed menstruation, possibly just an odd one and then menstruation resumes again for a month or two before another is missed. Gradually there are more missed menstruations than actual menstruations, but each menstruation lasts the expected number of days, say four to six days.

c) There is the sudden ending of menstruation, which had previously been regular, the final menstruation lasting the normal or nearly normal number of days. This abrupt ending is most likely if it has coincided with a stressful event, such as a daughter's wedding, moving house, or becoming a grandparent. This abrupt ending may even be the start of a depressive illness.

The individual woman's attitude to a missed or delayed menstruation depends upon her recent sexual activity and desire for pregnancy. If there has been no sexual activity she may not notice the infrequency or absence of menstrual bleeding for a month or two; but if the possibility of pregnancy exists her attitude changes to one of concern, with an increasing happiness or unhappiness as each additional day of missed menstruation passes and confirms the diagnosis. The possibility of pregnancy is usually uppermost in the minds of those whose regular menstruation suddenly ceases. While pregnancy is the commonest cause in the earlier years, one must always first consider the possibility of the menopause after 45 years of age. Comments by patients in this predicament include:

"I don't want to get my name in the *Guiness Book of Records* as the oldest Mother in the world."

"I would hate to be drawing my old age pension when my child is at school."

and from a grandmother:

"My child would then be younger than her niece."

Usually it is quite easy for a doctor to tell if a patient

is pregnant or undergoing the menopause. If she is pregnant her breasts will be full, she may have symptoms of early morning sickness and of passing urine during the night, and on examination her vagina is moist and the neck of the womb soft. On the other hand if she is entering her menopause her breasts will begin to decrease in size, she may have menopausal symptoms, especially flushes, and on examination her vagina will be pale and dry and the neck of the womb firm and smaller.

MENOPAUSAL FLUSHES

The most characteristic symptom of the menopause is the "hot flush," or "flash." It is a sensation of burning heat, arising from the waist and passing up to the top of the head. It only lasts a few minutes, five minutes at the most, and may be either visible, when the skin becomes flushed and beads of sweat appear, or it may be invisible. Very few women indeed pass through the menopausal years entirely without experiencing a single flush; they may range in frequency from only one or two a week to between fifty and a hundred a day. Many women are embarrassed by them, but others working with women of their own age giggle about them, believing that "a flush shared is a flush halved." Our grandparents used to say they were worth "a dollar a flush." They may be accompanied by palpitations, fluttering in the chest, or a feeling of choking, apprehension or anxiety. Flushes are worse immediately after a hot drink or spicy foods.

The flushes can occur at night, when the woman usually wakes abruptly in a bath of sweat; these are known as "night sweats." When the wife wakes suddenly flinging off the bedclothes, the husband is very likely to be annoyed rather than sympathetic.

A story is told about a group of women undergraduates at Girton College, Cambridge, in the twenties, who were discussing the menopausal problems and hot flushes that were being experienced by their parents and counselors. They agreed that as they were all so emancipated and fully understood the facts of life they would never have to suffer the ordeal of flushes. They formed a Menopause Club, promising to keep in touch with each other and give full accounts of how they fared through that great age. When the time came, each one of them experienced the flushes and other menopausal symptoms to a greater or lesser extent, in spite of their full knowledge of the events of life.

It would seem that the flushes are due to a sudden stimulus to the temperature controlling center in the hypothalamus, and are associated with a rise in the follicle stimulating hormone and luteinising hormone from the pituitary as well as a deficiency of estrogen.

MENOPAUSAL SYMPTOMS

The symptoms are usually divided into two groups. The specific symptoms, which are due to deficient estrogen and can be relieved by giving estrogen, and the vague psychological symptoms, some of which may be relieved by estrogen and some not, depending on the individual patient. Non-specific symptoms include tiredness, insomnia, irritability, depression, headaches, palpitations, anxiety, dizziness, forgetfulness and absentmindedness.

Lack of estrogen may cause the vagina to become dry, pale and thin which in turn may cause itching, pain or frequency in passing urine, often misdiagnosed as cystitis, pain on initial penetration at intercourse and ultimately loss of sex urge.

The skin becomes pale and thinner, it loses its elasticity so that wrinkles develop, especially on the face around the eyes and mouth, and in the neck. The soaring sales of cosmetics, beauty treatments and the demand for cosmetic surgery are evidence of the obvious distress caused by these middle age symptoms.

The rheumatic-like pains that develop in the bones, muscles and joints are due to the thinning of the bones. There is often marked stiffness on rising in the mornings, and the pains tend to move about from one site to another over the course of weeks. Sometimes the joints of the fingers may become very painful, with marked swelling, and then as the pain and swelling ease the joint may be left deformed and misaligned. In the postmenopausal years fractures of the wrist, neck of the femur and crushed fractures of the spine are a sign of marked thinning of the bones. The "dowager's hump" at the top of the spine is also a sign of thinning of the bones, but this does not develop until the seventies.

The thinning of the bones also causes a decrease in body height. Leonardo da Vinci in his "Universal Man" demonstrated that the height equals the armspan, and so it is for men and premenopausal women. However, as a woman's vertebrae become thinner after the menopause there is a decrease in height, with no corresponding decrease in armspan. If there is more than an inch and a half loss of height compared with armspan it is an indication that the woman should be on long term estrogen therapy. (Figure 30)

The worst symptoms are the non-specific ones which led to the following comments:

"I think I must be going insane."

"I feel so harassed the whole world seems to be resting on my shoulders."

"It's even tougher than pregnancy and labor."

At the menopause there are mood changes, which are continuous, not mood swings which last only two weeks or so at a time and are then eased, temporarily at least. It may turn an easy-going type into a shrew, a highly strung individual into a crying lunatic, a happy-go-lucky into an overworked, restless nagging bitch and a happy housewife into

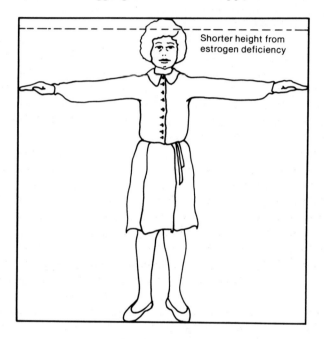

Shorter height from estrogen deficiency

Normally the armspan equals the height, but if estrogen deficiency occurs at the menopause the armspan exceeds the height

Figure 30   Relation between armspan and height

an absent-minded professor who puts the cat in the refrigerator and the milk on the doorstep. At this time the woman leaves the femininity rat-race and her personality factors become more important and possibly exaggerated.

Even the woman's shape alters as her breasts begin to

sag and she develops the spare tire and middle-aged spread. There is also the tendency for the thin to become even thinner and the fat to become obese.

DIAGNOSIS

The diagnosis is usually not difficult to make on clinical grounds. The hot flushes are most characteristic but it must not be forgotten that some anti-depressants can also cause flushes. The thin skin, the greying hair, the wrinkles, the dry vagina and deformed fingers and toes are all telltale signs. If further confirmation is needed a blood test will show a rise in follicle stimulating hormone and luteinising hormone, and if the bones are badly affected there will also be a rise in blood calcium and phosphates. A simple test which doctors can do is to examine some of the vaginal cells under a microscope; the cells with the ample estrogen have dark well-marked nuclei within them. This is known as the Karyopicnotic Index (or K. I.) and is often done routinely when a cervical smear is performed, but its value is limited to the times when progesterone is absent, such as just after a period and after a long interval since the last period. If progesterone is present the cells lose their nuclei.

If the diagnosis is in doubt it is worth giving the woman a month's trial of estrogen and if on her return she reports an improvement in the symptoms the prescription can be repeated. Admittedly there is frequently a beneficial placebo effect merely from giving the tablets, but if the benefit is still maintained two or three months later it strongly suggests that it is the hormone which is beneficial.

The effect of the menopause on sexual activity depends on one's experience during the menstruating years. If sex was important then it is likely to be even more enjoyable once the fear of pregnancy is permanently eradicated. If there was never much sexual excitement then many think of the menopause as a time when this activity may be slowed down or stopped. If estrogen deficiency is present and making the vagina sore and coital penetration painful these symptoms can be easily relieved by giving estrogen, either as a cream to be used locally or by tablets.

Those who talk and write, in error, of the "male menopause" refer to it as a time when a man's sexual urge diminishes. This is nothing more than anti-chauvinism. It is regrettable because it gives the impression that this is what is happening to women at the menopause, which is quite wrong.

When Neurgarten was carrying out his study on the attitude to the menopause he asked the loaded question "What is the best thing about the menopause?" to which 44% replied "not having to bother about menstruation," 30% "not being worried about getting pregnant" and 14% "a better relationship with husband and greater enjoyment of sex life."

The International Health Foundation in 1969 studied the subject and interviewed 2,000 women between 45 and 55 years and 72% agreed that after the menopause it was good to be free from menstruation. The figures for the various countries ranged from 66% in Italy to 79% in the United Kingdom.

EMPTY NEST SYNDROME

Unfortunately the menopausal years are often traumatic for women in other ways. It has been calculated that in the space of the five years around her fiftieth birthday, the average woman will lose her mother through death, her daughter through marriage and become a grandparent. There are also those whose children leave home for college or other employment, who move away or whose husband changes his job or receives his final promotion. This has led psychologists to refer to the "Empty Nest Syndrome," believing that all the miseries of the menopausal symptoms are but a reaction to the woman's empty life. While some women may be upset by these events, and accepting that such events will cause emotional impulses to reach the menstrual clock, nevertheless in the vast majority of cases the menopausal symptoms have a hormonal basis and respond well to estrogen therapy. Full details of treatment are to be found in Chapter 18.

17

Do It Yourself

There is a widespread hope that there may be some magic way of coping with monthly problems without having to disturb the busy doctor. Certainly in mild cases it is important to try to tackle the problems yourself, with the full knowledge that if you do not succeed further help, and the most effective help, is available from any doctor who understands hormone therapy.

First let us deal with the "old wives tales" and remind you that there's no truth in the idea that you mustn't have a bath, go swimming, or walk barefoot when you're menstruating or you will catch your death of cold. We now know that pneumonia commonly starts during the premenstruum, which is probably how the idea began. It won't matter if you do wash your hair when you're menstruating, although some women with very fine hair may find that a set at this time of the month won't stay in for long, so if you're paying for an expensive set wait just a few days longer. Another tale is that taking a cold shower will reduce the menstrual flow; this is wrong for the menstrual flow is going to come away normally in its own good time.

The desire to "do-it-yourself" came from a Community Nurse who wrote:

"I have always tended to be moody in my teens, but since

my second pregnancy I have spells of hell, during which my doctor gives me tranquilizers. These help a bit, but as a state-registered nurse and health visitor you can imagine my training screams out, 'Treat the cause, not the result.' Please tell me what I can do to help myself."

And from another nurse who pleaded:

"There must be something more – I don't just want to take anti-depressants permanently when I feel so very well and am perfectly O.K. for half of the month."

For those with spasmodic dysmenorrhea, relaxation and correct breathing is valuable, but unfortunately the benefit is not so marked in those with the premenstrual syndrome. It has been mentioned earlier that the type of pain suffered by those with severe spasmodic dysmenorrhea is similar to labor pains. Actually, the same nerves are involved in opening the door of the womb, to let the baby out, as are needed at menstruation to open the door to let out the menstrual flow. Nowadays it is universally recognized that in preparation for labor women benefit by relaxation exercises and correct breathing. Gradually it is being appreciated that these same relaxation exercises are of benefit to relieve the pain of dysmenorrhea. Some of our schools already teach their older girls relaxation as part of physical education and sufferers from dysmenorrhea have obtained much benefit from this. "Relaxation for Living" is an organization in Britain which exists purely to promote the teaching of relaxation, not only for that one day when the woman is in labor, but to help both men and women to relax during normal day-to-day living. They also have a cassette tape to help those who would prefer to learn relaxation in the coziness of their own home. The National Childbirth Trust runs classes throughout Britain for those who are pregnant, and are usually most helpful in supplying the name of a local teacher who will help either an individual or a group of girls with dysmenorrhea.

Drs. Margaret Chesney and Donald Tasto compared the effects of relaxation on college students in California. The students were initially separated into those with spasmodic dysmenorrhea and those with the premenstrual syndrome; they were then divided into one of three treatment groups by drawing lots. One treatment group received relaxation treatment at five weekly sessions and were told to practice the exercises daily at home, another group attended a leaderless psychotherapy group where they compared each other's experiences of period pain for five weekly sessions, and the last group were left untreated on the waiting list. All students completed questionnaires dealing with the severity of their pain before treatment and for three cycles after treatment was completed. Those who had spasmodic dysmenorrhea and took relaxation classes reported a dramatic improvement in their pain, which was sustained afterwards, but none of the other groups benefitted. So there does seem to be positive hope from simple treatment for those with spasmodic dysmenorrhea. However, if one is still being crippled with pain after thoroughly mastering the relaxation technique, there should be no hesitation in seeking help from the doctor, who can bring instant ease with a course of estrogen or prostaglandin inhibitors.

Sufferers from the premenstrual syndrome will need different help. The first important thing is to keep a menstrual chart. You can easily devise your own or use the types already described; it is the records which are important. If the chart shows the presence of symptoms during the paramenstruum with freedom of symptoms during another phase of the cycle, accept the diagnosis, realize you are not alone, but that some millions of other women are suffering likewise. Many letters received after a television program entitled

Pull Yourself Together, Woman expressed this sense of relief at knowing that they were not alone in their suffering:

> "I went to sleep happy that night knowing that I was not alone in my suffering."

> "Just to know I wasn't mad. I never dared talk about it, I thought I was the only one."

> "All my problems were so peculiar I didn't expect anyone else to understand."

What's more you might even try charting a friend's problems, such as colds, breakages, or temper tantrums. Some people have complaints month after month and never link it up or make the connection with menstruation, they merely announce "I've got another cold."

Having accepted the diagnosis yourself, talk about it. First your husband should know and understand so that he is able to help you. Wait until you feel well and then tell him how guilty you feel about your periodic loss of control, and if it is relevant, about your fears that you might one day harm your baby or attempt an overdose. As mentioned earlier, sometimes when you feel most down you nevertheless have an increased sex urge during the premenstruum. Discuss it with him, explain your difficulties, tell him that you know you're being horrid but you can't help it and you still love him and want him to love you. Having realized that there's nothing of which to be ashamed, talk to the other people with whom you come into contact so that they may be able to understand you better. Discuss it with your friends so that they can appreciate your difficulties and stand by you. Explain to your employer and to your in-laws, and don't forget it is just as important that men understand as well. Above all see that your adolescent children understand and accept all that it entails. If you are at school you should discuss it with your teacher, or if you are too shy you may like your mother to speak to the teacher instead.

During a Sunday family dinner my adolescent daughter broke a plate when she was clearing away the first course. "Don't worry, it's the wrong day of the month," commented my son. Not many minutes later my other daughter knocked over a glass and broke it. Trying to clear up the mess I knocked a bowl of vegetables onto the floor. "I think we men will have to take care of the washing up today," remarked my other son calmly. It seemed a far better way of dealing with a biological disturbance, rather than scolding the two girls for their apparent clumsiness and breakages.

Mark in your diary when you may expect your next period. Don't just count 28 days because others have a cycle of 28 days, but count the days of your last cycle and mark in the correct number of days for you personally. Consult your diary before arranging your next dinner party, avoid those awkward days if you have an interview, an examination or driving test. Arrange to have your permanent wave or tint during the postmenstrual week, it'll take better then. If you're a journalist don't accept a deadline for any article which will clash with the worst time of the month. School teachers in the high school can just as easily set homework two weeks ahead so that the girls can do it when in their postmenstrual peak. If you have to take examinations when you're feeling ill make sure you tell the proctor and he will write a note on your paper telling the examiner.

If you're at work tell your employer or your personnel manager. It helps if they understand. If flexitime is worked at your office you'll be able to keep some hours or days in hand to use when necessary. If there is shift work, try to get on the mid-day one, so that you've time to get up without hurrying and dose yourself up before starting the day's work. Sufferers from the premenstrual syndrome should, if possible, avoid night shift working as nothing is more unsettling for the menstrual clock than muddling night and day (remember the 'sleep and waking' control center is also in the hypothalamus near the menstrual clock). For the same reason, if you're going on a jet flight crossing the Atlantic be prepared to feel sleepy in the day and wakeful at night for a day or two after your journey.

In view of the importance of a fall in blood sugar level (discussed on pages 131–133), which can trigger off attacks of aggression, panics and migraine, it is worthwhile doing everything possible to prevent this happening. If you find you suddenly lose your temper, make a note of the time it happened (even if it wasn't your fault) and then write down all the times at which you have eaten food. Possibly you can do this together with your husband. If the result suggests the possibility of a long interval between food, make a determined effort to space your food out evenly throughout the day, rather than missing breakfast and relying on one full cooked meal in the evening. A snack at bedtime is helpful for those who have problems early in the morning. If you are dieting you can still divide your calories evenly into six snacks, there's no need to exceed the limit. If you are going to diet always start in the postmenstruum, never when your food craving is greatest and your weight highest during the paramenstruum. Unless you are being carefully supervised, do not attempt a crash diet or one relying on fluids only.

From ovulation onwards try to limit your fluids to four cups daily, there will always be enough liquid in your food which will be ample for your requirements. Strong coffee, not necessarily black, is a mild diuretic and may help to get rid of some extra water. If you're feeling very tired and lethargic make sure you've plenty of potassium-containing foods, such as bananas and tomatoes, or take some extra potassium tablets, which can be bought over the counter at drug stores.

If you're going to indulge in alcohol be warned that only half your usual amount will be required to make you merry. In sufferers from the premenstrual syndrome, intoxication can easily occur during the paramenstruum. It's as well to consider the other golden rules with regard to alcohol. Don't mix grape and grain alcohol, or better still don't mix your drinks. Avoid drinking on an empty stomach and don't drink and drive.

If you become constipated during the paramenstruum a dose of Epsom's Salts is probably the best laxative, as in addition to doing its job on the bowels it also removes water through the bowels which comes away with the feces.

It's a good idea to give yourself extra rest during the second half of the cycle, and if necessary an afternoon nap too. Even if you don't go off to sleep, or into a state of semi-consciousness, it is resting in bed in the dark with the eyes shut that counts.

If a sufferer from the premenstrual syndrome has taken all this advice and is still in trouble I would have no hesitation in suggesting a visit to the doctor, appreciating that he has help at hand specifically for your problem. But remember to take your carefully prepared chart with you so that he, too, can confirm the diagnosis.

Finally the menopausal woman, who is experiencing typical symptoms, would be well advised to avoid hot tea and coffee and spicy foods, in public anyway, as they do provoke the hot flushes. Try to diet carefully, remembering that during this phase of life it is very easy for the fat ones to get fatter and the thin ones to get thinner. Ensure a good night's rest, which is not necessarily the same as a good night's sleep, by avoiding too many blankets which will only encourage the night sweats. If the nights are very disturbed don't be ashamed of a short catnap after lunch. Your skin will also benefit from some cream to combat the natural dryness, and your greasy hair may need special shampoo.

18

What The Doctor Can Do

"How I resent those eight years of suffering now I know how easy it is to cure."

"If only others knew that operations and being admitted to hospital is not the answer to these beastly, savage changes of mood with the curse . . . the real treatment is so simple."

The first step the doctor has to take when seeing a patient with menstrual problems is to ascertain the diagnosis, reassure himself that there is not some other accompanying disease, such as depressive illness as well as premenstrual depression, and convince himself that there is no evidence of malignancy.

"My doctor treats all of us with a D & C and that's it."

This comment may well be true, and merely shows how careful the doctor is being in first eliminating the possibility of cancer in the body of the womb, which would not show up on a cervical smear or Pap smear. On the other hand, many gynecologists resort to the operation of dilation and curettage at the drop of a hat, and such treatment can do little enough to cure any hormonal imbalance.

Having made sure of his diagnosis the doctor now has

to decide whether to use hormone therapy and if so which one. In this book we have been concerned essentially with the two menstrual hormones, estrogen and progesterone. Earlier chapters have shown how a deficiency of either of them will result in a completely different presentation of symptoms. To give progesterone to a woman suffering from spasmodic dysmenorrhea or menopausal symptoms will only make her worse, and the same happens when estrogens are given for the premenstrual syndrome. This is why a definite diagnosis is essential before treatment can begin.

ESTROGEN THERAPY

The first estrogens to be used were non-steroidals, which had completely different formulas from the natural ones found in the body. These included stilbestral, dioenestral and hexoestradiol, which have been shown to have some cancer-producing potential and are rarely used today. The most important uses of estrogens are in the treatment of spasmodic dysmenorrhea, to help mature the womb in adolescence, at the menopause to substitute for the failing of the ovarian estrogen, and in the contraceptive pill.

SPASMODIC DYSMENORRHEA

In spasmodic dysmenorrhea the estrogen is given in courses from day 5 for 21 days, and menstruation usually occurs within two days. The first course will result in painless menstruation because it has stopped ovulation for that month, but if one wants to remove spasmodic dysmenorrhea permanently it is necessary to give many courses, perhaps for six to twelve months. In the sixties when doing an investigation into period pains it was surprising how many girls wrote that they had received one course of estrogens, which had only helped in that one month but made no difference thereafter. This is quite correct, but it is a shame it was not pointed out to the girls on starting treatment that more than one course would be necessary to remove pain altogether.

The estrogen can either be given alone or mixed with progestogens as in the estrogen-progestogen pill. The advantage of giving the pill is that one is sure menstruation will occur after 21 days and of course the pills are prepared in carefully dated packs of 21 so that they are not so easily forgotten, or if forgotten the mistake is easily visible and two tablets can be taken at once when remembered. On the other hand it can be treated by estrogen alone, in which case there is the advantage that varying strengths can be used; however bleeding does not always occur at the end of the course. If estrogen is used alone the girl must be fully aware that it is not a contraceptive.

> *Dierdre*, 19 years, had been given estrogen in Australia to relieve spasmodic dysmenorrhea. She came to Britain on a six-month holiday complete with sufficient tablets to last her stay. After about four months she realized she had missed her period and begun to develop morning sickness. Her pregnancy test proved positive.

As she was taking a pill every day for three weeks and stopping for one week, like all her friends who were on an oral contraceptive, she assumed hers was also contraceptive.

Mothers are often upset by the thought that their daughters are being given the pill to ease period pains; they need to be reassured and told that this will not immediately lead their virgin daughters up the path of rampant promiscuity. The girls too need to be reassured that in spite of the terrible pains their fertility is good, and the very fact of the pain shows that they are ovulating and so should not have much trouble in conceiving.

Occasionally women asking for treatment of spasmodic dysmenorrhea are also anxious to begin a family. In these cases it is worth giving a higher dose of estrogen from days 5 to 10 and days 18 to 28 of each cycle, avoiding estrogen at the time of ovulation so that conception can occur.

When estrogen is used for spasmodic dysmenorrhea before 25 years of age, side effects are rare because there is insufficient estrogen in the body and contraindications are hardly ever encountered.

Recently it has been shown that sufferers of spasmodic dysmenorrhea have a high level of a special substance known as "prostaglandin," which is produced by the disintegration of the lining of the womb shed at menstruation. This has provided a line of treatment for spasmodic dysmenorrhea using prostaglandin inhibitors. These tablets remove the pain and also reduce the amount of menstrual flow by about 25%. The tablets only need to be taken at the onset of menstruation and are continued for as long as the bleeding lasts. This treatment has the distinct advantage that it does not involve the use of estrogens and can be safely used by women who are trying to conceive.

ESTROGENS FOR MENOPAUSAL SYMPTOMS

When estrogens are given for menopausal symptoms the effect is dramatic. Within one week a marked lessening in the number of daily flushes may be expected, while if the flushes are still there in three weeks' time, it is a sign that a higher dose should be used. In Britain prescriptions for estrogens have increased by 50% during the last four years, suggesting that its value is now being fully appreciated.

Women who are still menstruating can have estrogen from day 5 until the time of their expected menstruation. While for many women this may mean a three week course, those with longer cycles would do better to have a longer course of estrogens, otherwise they may well have to go perhaps two weeks without treatment and risk the return of all their symptoms.

It is suspected that the build-up of the lining of the womb in women who are not menstruating may be so marked that it might predispose to a risk of cancer. No one really knows whether this is so, but there is a ready answer to this problem which is worth considering. The lining can be shed by the addition of some progestogen, taken for a few days and then stopped. Bleeding is then likely to occur within a day or two of stopping. The progestogen can either be added to the estrogen tablet and taken daily for three weeks and then stopped for a week during which bleeding will occur, or it need only be added for the last seven to ten days of the three weeks' course of estrogen.

On the other hand those women who have had the removal of their womb and are suffering from menopausal symptoms will also benefit from estrogen therapy. They will not need to have the added progestogen as there is no risk whatsoever of them developing cancer of the womb.

Estrogen can also be given by an implant, in which one or more small pellets of pure estrogen are inserted, under the influence of a local anesthetic, into the fat of the abdominal wall through a small incision in the skin. An implant means that the patient does not have the bother of trying to remember to take her daily tablets. It is particularly useful in women with menopausal symptoms who have had a hysterectomy in the past. An estrogen implant can also be performed for younger women during the course of their hysterectomy operation in order to prevent too great a shock to their menstrual hormonal pathway.

It is still a vexed question among the medical profession whether or not there is any risk in prolonged estrogen therapy. Certainly there does not appear to be a risk with short-term treatment. Follow-up studies of women, who have had estrogen for fifteen or more years, are difficult and confusing. In those days many women had the non-steroidal estrogens which are known to carry a risk. We only hear of the cases where cancer develops, and we do not know whether this really represents all the women in the sample who have been having estrogen for a long time. Even women who have never had estrogen do develop cancer of the womb. Several long term studies are in progress now, but it may be many years before the answer is available.

Women on estrogen therapy should be seen at least every six months for a check on their blood pressure and weight, and for a general examination and pap smear.

The side effects of estrogen are a feeling of nausea, bloatedness, headaches and depression, but these will only occur with women in whom there is no estrogen deficiency, such as women with the premenstrual syndrome.

At a recent meeting of a women's group where a talk was given on "Menopause" one member of the audience was very vocal and anxious to tell the audience that her doctor had refused to give her estrogen for her hot flushes. Later in the talk mention was made of the indications for avoiding estrogens, which include a past history of coronary thrombosis, angina, pulmonary embolism, deep vein thrombosis, cancer of the breast, womb or ovary, diabetes, liver disease and high blood pressure. The same woman then rose and apologized as she was under treatment for high blood pressure.

TREATMENT FOR THE PREMENSTRUAL SYNDROME

A woman journalist conducted a small private survey to find out what other doctors, up and down the country, were doing about menstrual problems. She noted the following as pretty standard answers.

> "It (progesterone) doesn't work, and anyway everybody's on the pill."

> "It can only be given by injections."

> "There is no proof it works."

> "Placebo effects."

> "Women are supposed to get some kind of masochistic pleasure from their pains."

There is nothing very surprising about these comments for they are typical of the attitudes which are delaying, for many many sufferers from the premenstrual syndrome, the relief to which they are entitled. The first one is typical of the confusion in many doctors' minds between progesterone and progestogens. Progestogens do not work on the pre-menstrual syndrome but progesterone does. The confusion is reinforced by the statement that follows, "everybody's on the pill." The next comment is from those who certainly know the difference but are unaware of the progress that has been made with suppositories and pessaries. The third re-mark is symptomatic of our scientific age which cannot accept the evidence of its own eyes without the support of strictly controlled trials. "The proof of the pudding is in the eating," or so it is said. The ladies whose quotes appeared at the beginning of this chapter needed no further proof of its value in treating the premenstrual syndrome than their own happy experience. The others need no comment and indeed they are all rather like doctors' old wives' tales. But in fairness to the doctors it must be remembered that very few who are practicing today were taught anything about these hormones when they were at medical school. However, there are also those doctors who do know how and when to use estrogen and progesterone to remove the monthly sufferings of women.

PROGESTERONE

The first time the word "progesterone" was used was by William Allen, who with George Corner first isolated the active constituent of the corpus luteum in the ovary. He proposed the name in December 1934 and eight months later the principal scientists involved in work on this new female sex hormone accepted the name. In 1943 Russell Marker emerged from the jungles of Central America and showed biochemists how to manufacture this pregnancy hormone, progesterone, from the roots of yams. However, once the biochemists had learned the knack of manufacturing progesterone from yams its importance was overshadowed by the many other steroids that could be obtained from progesterone just by a subtle alteration of its chemical formula. At their laboratories biochemists converted progesterone into the life-saving hormone, cortisone; it was also converted into progestogens, which are the basis of oral contraceptives and used by countless women the world over. (These synthetic progestogens are often mistaken for progesterone, but when taken by women they actually lower the progesterone level in the blood.) Progesterone is also converted into estrogens to satisfy the demand for hormone replacement therapy, and into testosterone for the restoration of male potency.

PROGESTERONE THERAPY

For many doctors progesterone is a forgotten hormone so far as treatment is concerned, and many doctors who use estrogen and know its possibilities and limitations are shy of using progesterone. One problem is that progesterone cannot be taken by mouth, as it is inactivated in the liver, so it has to be given in other ways. These include suppositories that can be inserted into the rectum or vagina, injections or implants. Recent work in India on monkeys has suggested that it is absorbed into the bloodstream when given by nasal administration, so who knows, we may yet be using it in aerosols, or nasal sprays.

When women with the premenstrual syndrome who have been treated with progesterone return to the doctor, it is often difficult to recognize them as the same women who first came for advice and treatment. The woman, who has so often taken an overdose during the late premenstruum when life was on top of her, will return delighted and must tell you of the interesting evening classes she is now attending. The alcoholic, who used to get herself into trouble each month, will discuss the dream holiday she is planning. The husband, who comes to tell you about his wife "who is now the woman I married." There is the mother who is so delighted because "even the children are behaving nowadays" and the student who has happily passed her final examinations, the epileptic mother whose children are once more returned home to her care and the asthmatic who drove to London Bridge to ceremoniously throw overboard her now redundant aerosol inhalers. For women who have suffered some of the serious consequences of the premenstrual syndrome that we have discussed in earlier chapters, it is really no hardship to have to administer their progesterone by pessary, suppository or injection, instead of the more conventional way through the mouth.

PROGESTERONE RECEPTORS

With advancing knowledge more is being learned about the way in which hormones are used in the body. Within many of the body cells are progesterone receptors whose task is to transport a single molecule of free progesterone from the fluid between the cells through the cell wall and the nuclear wall to the center of the nucleus where it is converted to use and later passes out of the body as pregnanediol. These progesterone receptors are in all parts of the body, but their concentrations are particularly in the brain, the eye, the nasal pharyngeal passages, the lungs, breasts, uterus and liver. It is the large concentrations in the liver which make oral progesterone ineffective for premenstrual syndrome. Anything taken by mouth goes via the portal system straight to the liver so, when progesterone is taken by mouth, it too will go straight to the liver where it is broken down. Therefore oral progesterone never reaches the systemic circulation and consequently does not get transported to the brain and other centers where it is needed. These progesterone receptors are very precise, they are created for progesterone and will accept only that, rejecting substitutes like the synthetic progestogens norethisterone, medroxyprogesterone, hydroxyprogesteronecaproate, dydrogesterone and all the contraceptive pills. This is the reason why synthetic progestogens are ineffective in cases of correctly diagnosed premenstrual syndrome.

PROGESTERONE SUPPOSITORIES

The progesterone suppositories are small pellets of inert wax containing progesterone. These are inserted in much the same way as tampons are inserted during menstruation. The wax melts at body temperature releasing the progesterone, which is absorbed through the lining of the vagina or rectum and conveyed in the blood to where it is needed. The wax is expelled from the body, either moistening the vagina or mixed with the feces. Women who have vaginal infection are invariably treated with suppositories and there are rarely any complaints. Suppositories are easy enough to insert into the anus, and were used by the ancient Egyptians, Greeks and Romans for the administration of drugs to the rectum, where they are easily absorbed into the bloodstream, but they have never been a popular method of treatment in Anglo-Saxon countries and America.

During a recent holiday in Spain we were enjoying a pleasant evening with our Spanish hosts when their four-year-old daughter emerged into the lounge complaining she couldn't go to sleep because of an earache. The mother searched in her handbag, gave the little one a suppository which she took away and apparently used herself quite satisfactorily. Women who have learned to appreciate the value of progesterone no longer object to using suppositories.

In practice rectal or vaginal suppositories are interchangeable and it is usually left to the individual which route she uses, or she can use both on alternate occasions. Patients are given permission to use an extra suppository when an unexpected need arises, such as when a sudden surge of irritability is building up or an impending migraine threatens. Up to four 400mg suppositories can be used in a day.

The time of giving progesterone will be determined by observing each individual patient's chart. In the normal case it is given as suppositories from midcycle until the onset of menstruation. However, if symptoms continue until the second or third day of menstruation then the progesterone should be continued until the fourth day. If symptoms start at ovulation the progesterone should be started a couple of days beforehand. In short there should be individual tailoring for each patient. The progesterone needs to be started at midcycle, or at least four days before the symptoms would be expected, thus it is useless to give progesterone suppositories on alternate days from day 19 to day 25 as was attempted in one controlled clinical trial.

The absorption of suppositories is quick and within twenty minutes there is a rise in the level of progesterone in the blood, but the progesterone level drops quite quickly too and the effect is always over within 24 hours while in some women the effect only lasts four hours. This means that some women need to take from two to six daily.

Progesterone injections last longer. In some women they only need to be repeated on alternate days, while others need them daily. The absorption is more reliable with injections and so they are used in desperate situations, such as when a marriage is at breaking point, or children are in danger of being taken into care. Another advantage is that if they are given daily by a district nurse she can silently supervise those who need watching in the premenstruum, for instance where there is a risk of suicide, child abuse or an alcoholic bout. Injections are more convenient for patients in hospitals and are also used where suppositories have failed.

At first the injections, which should be given deep into the buttock, are given by the practice, district or factory nurse, but with suitable instruction most patients soon learn the art of giving their own injections. Failing this the husband may be ready to learn the technique.

Progesterone can also be given by implants in those who have already had complete relief of symptoms with either suppositories or injections, as it relieves the need for daily medication and lasts for between six and eighteen months. It is particularly useful for women who have had a removal of their womb, as they will not be troubled by the erratic menstruation which sometimes occurs. It is also used for those who are forgetful in giving themselves progesterone, such as the feckless alcoholics. One patient living in Italy calculated that the cost of an annual implant, plus the air fare from Rome, was cheaper than the cost of daily suppositories.

However, a progesterone implant is not as convenient as an estrogen implant. More progesterone pellets are used and they sometimes have a tendency to be extruded, or pushed out. Attempts at extrusion are likely to occur at times of greatest progesterone need, such as during the premenstruum. The site of the implant becomes inflamed but can be eased by giving progesterone injections for five consecutive days, thus temporarily giving the body an alternative supply of progesterone.

A progesterone implant should not be given to those hoping to conceive within twelve months; those unduly concerned when their normal menstruation is replaced by an irregular scanty loss or possibly missed menstruation for spells of six months; those who must avoid premenstrual symptoms at all costs, such as the epileptic woman who may not appreciate her implanted supply of progesterone is running low and has an epileptic attack at a most unfortunate and potentially dangerous time; and those whose normal daily requirement of progesterone is very high.

If progesterone is given daily and then stopped for some reason menstruation will occur. This is similar to what happens when the level of progesterone drops and menstruation occurs in a normal cycle.

It is impossible to give an overdose of progesterone to a woman who has borne children, because during pregnancy women are exposed to a twentyfold increase in their blood progesterone level for nine full months, instead of just a mere two weeks, and the body has learned to deal with that. On the other hand, in childless and immature women an excess of progesterone may very occasionally cause euphoria and restless energy, insomnia and dysmenorrhea or uterine cramps similar to those suffered in spasmodic dysmenorrhea.

There are no contraindications for the use of progesterone. Also there are no risks of progesterone producing cancer, in fact progesterone is used in the treatment of some cancers, especially those produced in the vaginas of teenage girls who were exposed to stilbestrol (DES) during their fetal life, and also in treating advanced or recurrent cancer of the womb.

Progesterone suppositories in doses of 200mg and 400mg are commercially available in Britain under the trade name of "Cyclogest," manufactured by Messrs. L.D. Collins Ltd of Sunray House, 9 Plantagenet Road, New Barnet, Herts. For many years the Food and Drug Administration in the U.S. have permitted the commercial production of progesterone injections and also of 50mg progesterone suppositories for infertility patients with luteal phase deficiency of progesterone. Trials are now proceeding in the U.S. for the use of higher doses of progesterone. In Britain, progesterone suppositories of 200mg and 400mg have been available for 20 years and in my personal experience several thousand women have been using them for many years. Meanwhile, in the U.S. it is quite legal for any pharmacist to make up progesterone suppositories for any strength on a doctor's prescription for a named patient.

PROGESTOGENS

Because of the difficulty that progesterone cannot be given by mouth the biochemists sought for a synthetic preparation which could be absorbed orally. They tried making small alterations to the chemical formula hoping to find one with slightly different properties. After all, the formulae of estrogen, testosterone and cortisone are all very similar, although they have quite different properties. The biochemists succeeded in finding the progestogens, which are the basis of all contraceptive pills and gave rise to a multimillion dollar industry. When the progestogens were first discovered it was believed that they were true progesterone substitutes but in effect they had some properties of estrogen, some of progesterone and some of testosterone. If progestogens have been given during pregnancy and the child is a girl, she is likely to show masculinizing effects in her genitals and be a tom-boy with marked aggression. This is quite different from the effect of natural progesterone which is produced in such large quantities during pregnancy. Indeed surveys have suggested that if progesterone is given to mothers before the 16th week of pregnancy for eight weeks or longer, the child of that pregnancy has a tendency towards an enhanced intelligence, with a good academic record, higher grades and a better chance of reaching university level than control children whose mothers did not have progesterone. When a mother is taking a progestogen the level of her own progesterone in the blood is lowered. (Figure 31)

There are many differences between progesterone and the various progestogens, but unfortunately there are still some doctors who do not realize this. For instance progesterone can relieve water and sodium retention whereas some progestogens used in the pill, such as nor-ethisterone, cause a retention of water and sodium. Progesterone is converted by the adrenals into all the various corticosteroids, which is not possible with progestogens. The function of progesterone is also to maintain a pregnancy, but the progestogens cannot be used for this purpose. Some progestogens have an estrogenic effect as well, which is useful in the contraceptive field.

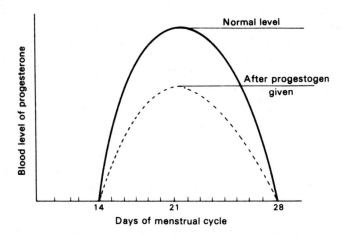

Figure 31   Effect of progestogen on the blood
level of progesterone

The usual progestogens in the pill cause a lowering of the blood progesterone level, and this is why women with premenstrual symptoms so often have difficulty in tolerating the pill whether it is the estrogen-progestogen or the progestogen-only pill.

CONTRACEPTION

For those who have or have had spasmodic dysmenorrhea,

the estrogen-progestogen pill is usually the best method of contraception. These women have a low estrogen level and benefit when given some extra estrogen, in fact many of these women were sorry when the high estrogen pills were removed from the market, as they said they felt so much better on a high dose. On the other hand the premenstrual syndrome sufferers are those who tend to have difficulty with the pill, causing an increase in headaches, gain in weight, depression and nausea, and these women are candidates for the more serious blood clotting problems. Furthermore the progestogens tend to lower the normal progesterone level making the premenstrual syndrome worse.

Unfortunately the intra-uterine devices have a tendency, in some women, to make menstruation heavier or longer, and therefore are best avoided in those who already have heavy periods.

Women who are having progesterone treatment for premenstrual syndrome can either take a progestogen-only pill from day 1 until day 11 and then start the normal progesterone dose until menstruation, or they can start with a small amount of progesterone from day 8, say a 50mg progesterone suppository, until their normal course of progesterone and continue it up to the start of menstruation. In this way they are contraceptively safe. Progesterone is Nature's own contraceptive, it is present after ovulation and converts the thin mucus into a thick, sticky type in which sperm cannot enter the womb.

Sterilisation is not the ultimate universal answer to contraception, for women with premenstrual syndrome may find the operation increases their symptoms (see page 20). Recently B.W. McGuiness, a family doctor in Cheshire, England, in a controlled series found that women who have bilateral tubal ligation suffered significantly more menstrual cycle disturbances post-operatively.

CONCEPTION

Those women on progesterone treatment who are anxious
to conceive are advised to start their progesterone 48 hours
after the temperature chart shows ovulation has occurred,
or if they do not know when ovulation occurs they should
start on day 16 for cycles of up to 28 days, and on day 18 for
longer cycles.

TESTOSTERONE

Testosterone, the male hormone, has occasionally been used
for the treatment of premenstrual syndrome, especially in
those who have sore breasts premenstrually. It is effective,
especially in giving energy and lightening or stopping menstruation, and easing the engorged breasts. However, it can
have masculinizing effects such as hoarseness, a deepening
of the voice, and the growing of hair on the beard area of
the face. Testosterone is also valuable in rapidly stopping
menopausal flushes and depression when it is given in a
combined tablet with estrogen. This may be useful for the
initial treatment for a month or two in a severely ill patient
at the menopause. Testosterone also improves the sex urge
and activity, and may be used in implants together with
estrogen.

BROMOCRIPTINE

Bromocriptine is a newly developed drug which is capable
of lowering a raised prolactin level. As explained in Chapter
14 sometimes a raised prolactin level interferes with the progesterone feedback pathway from the womb to the hypothalamus. There are reports from Holland that patients with infer-

tility and the premenstrual syndrome have been successfully treated with bromocriptine; however, strictly controlled trials on patients in England carried out by Ghose and Coppen, using a different dose, have not confirmed these findings. Patients who appear to benefit from bromocriptine are those with marked water retention, painful and engorged breasts, those who have lost their sex interest, those who have recently had a postnatal depression, and women with raised prolactin levels.

PYRIDOXINE

Pyridoxine, or Vitamin B6, is valuable in removing the depression that some women experience on the estrogen-progestogen pill and in menopausal women on estrogen therapy. It has been tried, but not successfully, for the treatment of premenstrual syndrome, in which it appears helpful in the milder cases of depression, but not for physical symptoms.

CLONIDINE

Clonidine, marketed in the United Kingdom under the name of Dixarit, is a drug for the lowering of blood pressure, and in very small doses it may be used to relieve menopausal flushes in those who for some reason are unable to tolerate estrogens. However, it only acts on the flushes and is of no value in relieving the other estrogen-deficiency symptoms at the menopause, such as vagina and skin thinning, joint pains and the psychological symptoms. One beautiful menopausal lady, who always had a perfectly coiffured head of white hair, refused to have a further course of estrogens, which although they cured her menopausal flushes and depression caused some of her white hairs to become grey again. She opted for Clonidine, at least for a few months until the psychological symptoms bore down on her.

DIURETICS

It is best to avoid diuretics as any help they give to those with water retention is only temporary, and it is so easy to repeat them indefinitely, always taking more and more until the balance of sodium and potassium is disturbed. Diuretics do not help the premenstrual tension, depression or irritability, only the symptoms due to water retention, such as bloatedness, gain in weight and swollen ankles.

POTASSIUM

A lowering of the blood potassium level may be suspected in those who have been taking diuretics for a long time, those who have food cravings and prolonged dieting and those who complain of exhaustion and muscle weakness throughout the cycle. These women should have a blood potassium estimation, and if necessary be given potassium tablets regularly.

19

A Fairer Future

This book was written with the aim of spreading the news to mankind that the once-a-month miseries of countless women can be, and are being, successfully relieved and treated. At the same time it was hoped that it would help men to understand and appreciate the menstrual problems of women and become partners in helping them through those difficult days. That you are reading this brings hope that the aim will be achieved.

The menstrual miseries are widespread and incapacitating at times; their effects can involve all classes and all ages and both sexes. Nevertheless it is possible to abolish dysmenorrhea, the premenstrual syndrome and menopausal problems by hormone treatment. But although treatment is possible it is not yet universal. Menopausal clinics are now well established and countrywide gynecological help is available for the relief of symptoms related to the change of life. The recognition of premenstrual syndrome is not yet as widespread, although since the first edition of this book there have been some encouraging finds. For a list of clinics, support and information groups, see Appendix II, p. 217.

The premenstrual syndrome really should be a speciality of general practice, and should be mastered by every general practitioner. The day will surely come when every general practitioner and consultant is able to diagnose, treat and manage all cases of the premenstrual syndrome which come within their orbit. At present this goal is a long way off.

The gynecologist tends to be satisfied with a faultless physical examination and the reassurance of a "D & C" and is then content to refer the patient back to the family doctor. The endocrinologists have more serious diseases to occupy their time and rarely wish to be troubled by disturbances of menstrual hormones, especially at a time when there are not enough useful hormonal estimations to clinch the diagnosis and determine the dose of hormones needed. Psychiatrists do occasionally recognize the syndrome, prescribe anti-depressants or tranquilizers, but then see the patient in the symptom-free postmenstruum and discharge her from their care. The neurologists fully investigate all cases of epilepsy and migraines to satisfy themselves no lesion is present and discharge the patient. The chest physician treats the asthma, the rhinologist the allergic rhinitis, the orthopedic surgeon and rheumatologist the backache and painful joints, the dermatologists the herpes and neuro-dermatitis, but even if all the menstrually-related symptoms are appreciated by these consultants, the diagnosis is still too easily ignored.

If Premenstrual Syndrome Clinics are to be established the general practitioner will need to be in the forefront, assisted by a psychiatrist and gynecologist, for it is only the general practitioner who encompasses the whole vista of symptoms and knows the effect on the family. Before he is ready to accept his role the general practitioner needs specialized courses in diagnosing and treating these menstrual problems, and medical students require a greater familiarity with the subject during their undergraduate training. The general practitioner needs to know the art of adjusting menstruation for vital events, knowing the hazards and methods, the utilization of the peak postmenstrual days and recognizing the women with dysmenorrhea and premenstrual syndrome who urgently need treatment.

The need for greater public education and awareness is obvious, and here is an opportunity to be grasped by the media and offered to a public always hungry for human stories of medical possibilities, but we must remember that doctors do not like to be told by the popular press what treatment they should give their patients. Education on these subjects should extend to schools, where both sexes should be made aware of the problems and the solutions which are at hand.

It is estimated that the cost of menstrual problems to American industry is equal to 8% of the total wage bill. Would it not be better for industry to invest a fraction of that sum in menstrual clinics and training schemes for doctors, in order to speed the time when such wastage will be eliminated?

School and university examinations can be made fairer by adjusting the timetable so that exams are set a week apart, by having compulsory questions in all tests rather than one compulsory exam, by setting alternative dates where possible, and by offering a choice of dates for practical and oral examinations. Teachers can set the pupils work two or more weeks in advance.

A greater appreciation of the relationship of the premenstrual syndrome to violence and battering would enable premenstrual baby battering to be correctly diagnosed, understood and treated, thereby eliminating the problem and removing the social stigmas of separation, children being taken into care and criminal proceedings.

The ideal would seem to be to abolish menstruation altogether at those times when conception is not required. Already this is possible by the prolonged administration of progestogens, but not yet ideal. Initially there tends to be the occasional breakthrough bleeding, and then after a year or two there is a subtle change in the personality of the woman: she becomes harder and more efficient, with loss of sex interest. Is the price worth it? Already there is the technique of menstrual aspiration which women can learn to perform themselves, in which they suck the menstrual flow from the womb through a thin flexible plastic tube and complete menstruation in one minute or less. Unfortunately menstrual hormones may be upset by this event and their smooth ebb and flow drastically altered. The layman, or rather laywoman, too eagerly hopes that the mere removal of the womb will accomplish the feat, but as has already been discussed the removal of the womb too often upsets the hormonal pathway and the end result may be worse than before the operation.

In the last century John Ruskin reminded his fellow countrymen that "the true wealth of the Nation was running to waste" because most children had no sort of education. The same could be said today about the lack of education and understanding of the premenstrual syndrome. The discussion of menstruation and its attendant problems should be as open and unrestricted as the discussion of sex, and the knowledge and understanding of menstruation should be available to all.

Having read as far as this, there will probably be two questions nagging at your mind. "If progesterone and estrogen are so successful in their respective treatments, why are there not more doctors using them?" and "Why do some doctors prefer to use a drug which is less successful and only brings partial relief to a portion of patients with mild symptoms, rather than one which brings complete relief to most patients with mild and severe symptoms?"

There is no simple answer to these perfectly reasonable questions. Some answers are contained in earlier chapters, but there are a number of other reasons which can be roughly grouped under four broad headings:

1) Doctors have an essentially conservative approach.
2) The spread of information.
3) Commercial aspects.
4) Lack of consultancy and treatment facilities.

Very few of the doctors in practice today had any training in diagnosing or treating what we now know is the world's commonest disease, the premenstrual syndrome. Doctors are themselves wholly responsible for the diagnosis and treatment of their patients and they alone have the right to protect their patients as well as themselves, and therefore have a natural reticence to using treatments which they personally are not yet fully persuaded are safe and effective.

This leads us to the spread of information, for how is the doctor to learn about new treatments and new drugs? Medical journals have limited space and take time to read and many of the articles do not necessarily concern the general practitioner. Most of his information is obtained from the representatives of the drug companies who regularly visit him. The drug companies are commercial concerns with products to sell and so the doctor is kept persuasively aware of the value of treatments. Some drug companies spend vast sums of money on research into new drugs, not merely in the interest of the patient but with an eye to the potential financial return. Recently one or two of them have embarked on financing treatment for menstrual problems. As the patent rights for progesterone ran out a long time ago no large pharmaceutical company is particularly interested in marketing a product that does not give them an exclusive market. No commercial firm is going to gain financially by advertising progesterone for the premenstrual syndrome.

The general practitioner, who has a patient with a condition he does not understand, will forward that patient to a consultant who specializes in that particular problem.

But to whom will he send the premenstrual asthma or the premenstrual sinusitis which has been confirmed by a menstrual chart? Not to a gynecologist or endocrinologist or psychiatrist. This is why there is a great need for more Premenstrual Syndrome Clinics.

These are but partial answers to those questions, but it must be appreciated that all the time the number of doctors who can diagnose and treat these menstrual problems increases month by month. If more clinics could be established and training courses instituted the number of undiagnosed and untreated sufferers would steadily decrease.

A quotation by Henry David Thoreau runs:

> "If you have built
> Castles in the air,
> Your work need
> Not be lost;
> There is where they
> Should be.
> Now put foundations under them."

Let us get down to work.

Other Publications by the Author

The Premenstrual Syndrome (1953) Joint authorship R. Greene. Brit. Med. J., 1, 1007.

The Premenstrual Syndrome (1955), Proceedings of the Royal Society of Medicine, 48, 5, 337.

Menstruation and Acute Psychiatric Illnesses (1959), Brit. Med. J., 1, 148.

Effect of Menstruation on Schoolgirls' Weekly Work (1960), ibid., 2, 1425.

Menstruation and Accidents (1960), ibid., 2, 1425.

Menstruation and Crime (1961), ibid., 2, 1752.

The Influence of Menstruation on Health and Disease (1964). Proc. Roy. Soc. Med., 57, 4, 262.

THE PREMENSTRUAL SYNDROME (1964), London: William Heinemann Medical Books.

The Influence of Mother's Menstruation on her Child (1966) (Charles Oliver Hawthorne, BMA Prize Essay), Proc. Roy. Soc. Med., 59, 10, 1014.

The Influence of Menstruation on Glaucoma (1967) Charles Oliver Hawthorne, BMA Prize Essay), Brit. J. Ophthal., 51, 10, 692.

Ante-Natal Progesterone and Intelligence (1968), Brit. J. Psych., 516, 114, 1377.

Menstruation and Examinations (1968), Lancet, 11, 1386.

THE MENSTRUAL CYCLE (1969), Penguin Books.

Children's Hospital Admissions and Mother's Menstruation (1970), Brit. Med. J., 2, 27–8.

Migraine in General Practice (Migraine Trust Prize Essay) (1973), J. Royl.Coll. Gen. Pract., 23, 97.

Effect of Progesterone on Brain Function (1975), X Acta Endocrin. Congr., Amsterdam.

Sexual and Menstrual Problems in the Blind (1976), Conference of Sexual Problems of the Disabled. Royal College of Obstetricians and Gynaecologists, London.

Migraine and Oral Contraceptives (1976), Headache, 15, 4, 247.

Prenatal Progesterone and Educational Attainments (Charles Oliver Hawthorne Prize 1976), Brit. J. Psych., November, 129, 438.

THE PREMENSTRUAL SYNDROME AND PROGESTERONE THERAPY (1977) London: William Heinemann Medical Books Ltd., and Chicago: Year Book Medical Publishers Inc.

Cyclical Criminal Acts in Premenstrual Syndrome (1980), Lancet, 1070–1071.

DEPRESSION AFTER CHILDBIRTH (1980) Oxford University Press.

The Legal Implications of Premenstrual Syndrome (1982) World Medicine, 17th April 1982.

Glossary

Adrenal glands – two glands situated above the kidney and responsible for producing numerous hormones.

Adrenalin – one of the many hormones produced by the adrenal glands.

Analgesics – pain relievers.

Ante-natal – before childbirth.

Anovular – without ovulation.

Cervical smear – test for the diagnosis of cancer of the neck of the womb.

Cervix – neck of the womb.

Climacteric – change of life.

Corticosteroids – hormones produced by a part of the adrenal glands.

Diuretics – drugs capable of increasing the amount of urine passed.

Dysmenorrhea – pain with menstruation.

Endometrium – inner lining of the womb.

Estrogen – hormone produced by the ovaries.

Fallopian tubes – two tubes leading from the ovaries to the womb, along which the egg cells pass.

Geriatrics – care of the elderly.

Glaucoma – disease of the eye characterized by raised pressure in the eye ball.

Gynecology – study of the diseases of the woman.

Hormones – chemicals produced by glands, which pass in the bloodstream to exert an action at a distant site.

Hypothalamus – specialized part of the base of the brain concerned with control of metabolism.

Hysterectomy – surgical removal of the womb.

Implant – pellets of drugs inserted into the tissue.

Intermenstruum – part of the menstrual cycle not covered by the premenstruum or menstruation, usually days 5 to 24.

Intra-uterine device – small contraceptive appliance inserted into the womb.

Menarche – first menstruation.

Menopause – last menstruation marking the end of the childbearing era.

Menstrual clock – the specialized portion of the hypothalamus responsible for the cyclical timing of menstruation.

Menstrual cycle – time from the first day of menstruation to the first day of the next menstruation.

Menstrual loss – bleeding at menstruation.

Menstruation – monthly bleeding from the vagina in women of childbearing age, caused by the disintegration of the lining of the womb.

Metabolism – building up and breaking down of chemicals in the body.

Migraine – severe form of headache.

Mittelschmerz – abdominal pain at the time of ovulation (middle pain).

Ovary – reproductive organ containing the egg cells.

Ovulation – release of the egg cell from the ovary.

Ovum – egg cell.

Paramenstruum – premenstruum and menstruation.

Pituitary – gland situated at the base of the brain and controlling many other glands.

Postmenstruum – the days immediately after menstruation.

Post-natal – after childbirth.

Premenstruum – the days immediately prior to menstruation.

Pre-ovulatory –days before ovulation.

Progesterone – hormone produced by the ovary for the preparation of the lining of the womb. Also a starting point for the production of numerous corticosteroids.

Progestogen – synthetic drugs used in contraceptives, once thought to be a progesterone substitute.

Prolactin – hormone produced by the pituitary gland.

Puerperium – after childbirth.

Spasmodic dysmenorrhea – spasms of pain occurring with menstruation.

Synchrony – at the same time.

Syndrome – collection of symptoms which commonly occur together.

Testosterone – male hormone.

Therapy – treatment.

Uterus – womb.

Vagina – passage leading from exterior of the body to the mouth of the womb.

APPENDIX I

PMS: The Need for Legal Guidelines and Accurate Diagnosis

It was a surprising coincidence that on consecutive days, two women in different English cities appeared in court charged with murder. Both charges were reduced to manslaughter on the grounds of diminished responsibility caused by premenstrual syndrome. Although the circumstances of their offenses were quite different, the evidence presented in each case led to the same conclusion: each defendant was suffering from a severe case of premenstrual syndrome. Both cases had been very carefully researched and presented incontrovertible evidence of longstanding, bizarre, cyclical behavior occurring in the premenstruum with normality of behavior in the postmenstruum. The important point to appreciate is that these were two extreme and exceptional cases.

The definition of premenstrual syndrome is *"the presence of recurrent symptoms in the premenstruum or early menstruation with a complete absence of symptoms after menstruation."* Thus if a plea of premenstrual syndrome is put forward there must be evidence of recurrent symptoms, or earlier episodes of a similar loss of control, confusion, amnesia or violence in previous cycles, or at monthly intervals. Such evidence found in diaries, medical records, police files, prison documents, might give the precise dates of marital quarrels, physical violence, previous suicide attempts or slashing of the wrists.

An 18-year-old ballet dancer accused of arson successfully pleaded premenstrual syndrome as a mitigating factor and was released on probation. She had an excellent school report and her behavior was exemplary until menstruation started, at which time she appeared to change in character and started episodes of unusual and unexplained behavior. One day she suddenly went into her bedroom and shaved off her blonde hair and eyebrows; on another occasion she ran away from home and was later returned by the police having been found drunk and disorderly; once she burned her bedroom curtains; another time she overdosed herself with pain relievers and alcohol and was admitted to hospital overnight; finally she set fire to her father's house and was admitted to prison. While in prison she attempted to set fire to the bed in her cell, and on another occasion she attempted to strangle herself by tying one end of her sheet around her neck and the other end to the top of the window. It was her father who noticed from his diaries that his daughter's problems occurred about once a month. He was advised to produce proof of the precise dates on which the many curious happenings occurred. There followed a search through the doctor's and hospital's files, dates of insurance claims for the burnt curtains, the date on the check on which he bought his daughter a new wig, and the precise dates on which she misbehaved while in prison. Again the many occurrences were shown to be coming in regular monthly cycles. She received progesterone treatment and is now a normal well-behaved woman.

A similar story can be told of an unemployed girl who harassed the police with unnecessary emergency phone calls. Earlier she had been in a reform school for such phone calls, but on release the emergency phone calls persisted and disrupted normal police work. She was imprisoned. Her father again was the one who noticed that the problems arose each month and drew the lawyer's attention to the coincidences. In her case it represented a cry for help, akin to other women whose cry for attention may take the form of slashing their wrists. She too responded to progesterone and was released on probation. However, on her return to civilian life progesterone was not restarted and she again made unnecessary phone calls to the police. This time no mercy was shown and she served a two year sentence. She is now once more at liberty, but taking progesterone treatment regularly.

These represent genuine cases of criminal behavior resulting from a hormonal disease which responded to treatment. These women should rightly be freed for they cannot be held responsible for their sudden unexpected loss of control. However, the genuine cases are few and far between. A far bigger problem has now arisen and it is our duty to ensure that premenstrual syndrome is not made a universal defense. Already cases have occurred in Britain where this has been tried. A woman on her first charge of shoplifting cannot make a claim of premenstrual syndrome without evidence that this is a recurrent offense. The mere coincidence of two car crashes, or two speeding offenses occurring in the premenstruum is insufficient evidence of premenstrual syndrome. The public has a right to be protected by the knowledge that the defendant is receiving progesterone treatment and is unlikely to be a further danger. At a recent appeal trial in Britain premenstrual syndrome as a defense in a case of murder was rejected although it still stands as a "factor causing diminished responsibility" in capital charges and as "a mitigating factor" in lesser charges.

For the correct diagnosis of premenstrual syndrome, the precise dates of menstruation and of the alleged crime are a prerequisite. Yet a clerk in a travel agency, accused of stealing travelers' checks worth $1,000 from her employer at some unknown date between August 1980 and April 1981, pleaded premenstrual syndrome. Not surprisingly the plea failed and a jail sentence was imposed.

Some women are needlessly incarcerated because of premenstrual syndrome. They are deserving of our sympathy, and justice will not be served until all true sufferers of premenstrual syndrome are properly diagnosed and treated.

To summarize,

1) Because of recent findings on PMS, it becomes necessary to recognize this disease as a factor in criminal behavior in women.
2) It is also necessary to form a clear legal understanding of the meaning of PMS. This is important because of an inevitable abuse of the law by criminals.
3) It is also important to point out that this does not mean all sufferers of PMS are potential murderers, nor does it mean all female murderers suffer from PMS.
4) PMS is only a contributing factor to the case and should be taken in consideration with other evidence.
5) PMS is a real hormonal/organic/physiological disorder and should not be overlooked as trivial, for this would be an injustice to the sufferer.

In the following papers some of these arguments and evidence are covered in more detail. These papers were previously published in medical jouranls and are reproduced here for the serious reader and to help medical and legal researchers.

(The original style and spelling of the English publication has been retained in these following reprints.—*Ed.*)

LEGAL IMPLICATIONS OF PMS

(Reprinted from World Medicine, April 1982)

A new responsibility has been placed on the medical profession as a result of the recent legal rulings recognising premenstrual syndrome (PMS) as a cause of diminished responsibility in two women charged with manslaughter. **It now becomes our**

duty to ensure that the plea of PMS will not be abused. To do this will require that in every case the diagnosis of PMS is substantiated with incontrovertible evidence and that it will respond to treatment. Only the doctor can provide such evidence and ensure that the diagnosis is not abused.

Those few women who lose control of themselves for a day or two, month after month, need help and help is available. However, they must not be confused with the other 99.9 per cent of women who are well able to control their actions. PMS is not a universal defence, nor should it be allowed to become one. Medical evidence is required by the court and the doctor must become fully conversant with the recognition, diagnosis and treatment of the syndrome.

More than 30 years of research into PMS has produced a clear and precise definition: "the presence of *monthly recurrent* symptoms in the premenstruum or early menstruation with a *complete absence* of symptoms after menstruation." The words "monthly recurrent" and "complete absence" are essential in every correct diagnosis and the symptoms should have recurred in at least three consecutive menstrual cycles.

Furthermore, it must be borne in mind that at the PMS clinic at University College Hospital, London, the diagnosis of PMS is confirmed in only half of the women claiming to have PMS. This is a similar figure to that noticed by Dr. Ronald Norris at the PMS Clinic in Boston, Mass.

The presence of "recurrent symptoms" implies that when a woman makes a plea of PMS at her first offence, that plea fails unless she can produce positive evidence of similar episodes of loss of control, confusion, amnesia or violence in the three previous cycles. Such evidence might be supplied by her employers, friends or family, or by searching through diaries, medical files, police records or prison documents.

The three cases of cyclical criminal charges in PMS reported in the *Lancet* in 1980(1) had been scrupulously researched. Indeed the woman charged with manslaughter had 30 previous convictions, occurring at cycles of 29.04 ± 1.47

days, and even while in prison had 26 episodes of bizarre behaviour including attempted strangling, drowning, attempted escape, slashing wrists, smashing windows and setting fire to her cell. These episodes, so meticulously documented by the prison officers on duty, occurred at intervals of 29.55 ± 1.45 days. The diagnosis did not rely on the woman's memory. Furthermore she was described as "pleasant and cooperative but at times she loses her senses and can be quite impulsive," which suggests that there was a complete absence of destructive symptoms after menstruation.

In contrast there is the case of a 22-year-old driver who made a successful plea at Burnham, Bucks, that PMS was the cause of her dangerous driving, as both crashes occurred within 48 hours of menstruation. She was not asked for additional evidence of any lapses of concentration in previous premenstruums, nor evidence of exemplary alertness in the postmenstruum. The occurrence of two crashes in the premenstruum could have been a mere coincidence.

In 1977 a 46-year-old part-time social worker faced a charge of shoplifting. In evidence she produced her diary showing the days of confusion each month, when she refused to leave the house, and she arranged her days at work accordingly. Her husband had recognised these cyclical occasions of confusion and described how she would return home from shopping with dog food, although they kept no animals, or a child ski outfit although their own children were now adult. Together with his wife, they had marked in the diary the days on which trouble might occur. All was well until a member of the staff caught the 'flu and the social worker agreed to alter her working days. The case was dismissed. She has since received progesterone treatment and been free from these lapses of concentration and confusion.

For a correct diagnosis of PMS the precise dates of menstruation and of the alleged crime are essential. A clerk in a travel agency was accused of stealing travellers cheques worth

$1000 from her employer at some *unknown date* between August 1980 and April 1981. Her plea of PMS failed.

There are certain features which are characteristic of the offences committed by sufferers of PMS, which may be easily recognised.

1. The woman acts alone without an accomplice.
2. The offence is not premeditated, and usually comes as a surprise to those whom she was with shortly before the event.
3. The action is without apparent motive, such as setting fire to an unknown person's property.
4. There may be no attempt to escape detection. A woman randomly throwing a brick at a shop window may herself telephone the police and await her arrest.
5. The action may be *cri de coeur*, as with the hoaxer who repeatedly makes emergency 999 calls. This is similar to a parasuicide.

Among the more frequent symptoms of PMS which may result in criminal charges are a sudden and momentary surge of uncontrollable emotions resulting in violence, confusion or amnesia, alcoholism, nymphomania and attention-seeking episodes which represent cries for help. These cover a full range of criminal offences such as actual violence, damage to property, theft and disorderly behaviour.

Sufferers of PMS characteristically have painfree menstruation. The shoplifter, who claimed her period pains were so severe that she was under the influence of pain-relieving drugs at the time of her offences, was suffering from spasmodic dysmenorrhoea and not from PMS. Incidentally, each of the three women reported in the *Lancet* was referred for a diagnosis of PMS by her father, who had noticed that his daughter's unpredictable behaviour occurred every four weeks. The three offenders had painfree menstruation and had not themselves associated this cyclical physiological event with their strange behaviour.

A full medical history will reveal many characteristic features, which confirm or refute the diagnosis. The onset of PMS, and the occasions of increased severity, always occur at times of hormonal upheaval, as at puberty, during or after taking the Pill, after amenorrhoea, pregnancy or sterilisation. These are the women who have side-effects on the Pill, and their pregnancy may be complicated by pre-eclampsia or postnatal depression.(2) During the premenstruum they have difficulty in tolerating long intervals without food (over five hours daytime or 13 hours overnight) and they become easily intoxicated by alcohol in the premenstruum.

A 32-year-old Essex housewife was accused of infanticide, having drowned her second daughter and then overdosed herself. She started menstruating in the intensive care unit and mention of PMS was noted in her previous medical records. She had developed migraine and hypertension on the Pill, for which she was admitted for observation to the London Hospital. Her first pregnancy was complicated by pre-eclampsia and after her second pregnancy she developed postnatal depression requiring a psychiatric domicilliary visit. The incident occurred about 5:30 pm; she had no food since her 8:30 am breakfast. The court accepted the several diagnostic pointers of PMS and she was released on probation and treatment.

Among PMS women, increased libido is occasionally noticed in the premenstruum, a fact recorded by Israel back in 1938. All too often it is this nymphomanic urge in adolescents which is responsible for young girls running away from home, or custody, only to be found wandering in the park or following the boys. These girls can be helped, and their criminal career abruptly ended with hormone therapy.

Treatment with progesterone (*not* synthetic progestogen)

is effective in well diagnosed cases of PMS, but not in menstrual distress, which is a term covering a multitude of disorders, including spasmodic dysmenorrhoea, endometriosis, hyperprolactinaemia, pelvic inflammatory disease, and symptoms of other diseases present through the cycle, but exacerbating during the paramenstruum, e.g., depression, neurosis, psychosis, migraine, arthritis, bronchitis.

Menstrual distress may be diagnosed by the use of the Moos Menstrual Distress Questionnaire (MMDQ) but this cannot be used for the diagnosis of PMS as it was not designed to reveal the recurrence of symptoms in the premenstruum or the absence in the postmenstruum, nor does it do so.

It is estimated that one in 10 of all menstruating women suffer from PMS severe enough to deserve treatment, but the proportion of sufferers charged with criminal offences is unknown. Some PMS women are needlessly detained and deserving of sympathy, and justice will not be done, or seen to be done, until the true sufferers are diagnosed and treated. PMS has been trivialised by the media and feminine interests will best be served by our ability to distinguish the few genuine sufferers from the many malingerers whose claims can never be substantiated.

REFERENCES
1. Dalton K. *Lancet* 1980;2:1070.
2. Dalton K. *Premenstrual Syndrome and Progesterone Therapy.* William Heinemann Medical Books, London, 1977.

THE IMPORTANCE OF DIAGNOSING PREMENSTRUAL SYNDROME

(Reprinted from **Health Visitor**, February 1982)

Introduction

In the 1950s, doctors were urged to look afresh at their chronic patients to ensure that they were not suffering from hidden depression which would respond to the newly discovered anti-depressants. Now, with our improved understanding of pre-menstrual syndrome (PMS), there is a similar need to take a new look at those chronic problem patients who are women in their menstruating years. We need to see whether they are victims of PMS who are suffering needlessly when they could be given the benefit of the highly successful treatment with natural progesterone.

Recently, premenstrual syndrome has been given legal recognition as a cause of diminished responsibility in murder, and as a mitigating factor in crimes of arson, assault, shoplifting and disorderly conduct. However, the law requires more than the mere statement that the woman was in her premenstruum at the time of her crime. Evidence must be produced to show that the symptoms recur regularly each month, and that treatment is likely to be successful and ensure that she will not repeat the offence.

Characteristics of PMS

Premenstrual syndrome is a disease of progesterone deficiency. The symptoms of PMS will therefore only occur in the second half of the menstrual cycle when adequate amounts of progesterone in the peripheral blood are required. After menstruation and until ovulation, progesterone is not present in the peripheral blood and so PMS symptoms will not occur. Therefore it follows that for the diagnosis of PMS it is essential to show that the timing of symptoms is limited to the premenstruum or early menstruation, with a complete absence of symptoms after menstruation. Diagnosis is best achieved by use of a menstrual chart on which the woman marks with an "M" the dates of menstruation (or with a "P" the dates of her period), and then uses other symbols for her symptoms, for example "X" for the days of quarrels, alcoholic bouts or asthma attacks, "T" for tiredness, "F" for forgetful days and "H" for headaches. Each woman can select symbols for her most troublesome symptoms. Charts are obtainable free from Cox-Continental Ltd, Brookside Avenue, Rustington, Sussex. Diagnosis rests on ensuring that there is a complete absence of symptoms during the postmenstruum. With a menstrual chart this diagnosis can be made at a glance, in fact even a ten-year-old child can recognize those charts which have no symbols for at least seven days after the "M"s.

Interviews with husbands and parents are invaluable, as those closest to the PMS sufferer will know best how she changes from the happy, charming individual which she is on most days into the lazy, irritable and unpredictable female she becomes as menstruation draws near.

Retrospective Diagnosis

In order to obtain a retrospective diagnosis it may be helpful to conduct searches elsewhere. Looking up the school register may reveal a monthly pattern of school truancy, as occurred in one teenager who was frightened to go to school on those days when his mother hit the bottle. Hospital records will show the precise dates of overdoses and self-mutilation attempts. The work register may be consulted to show cyclical absences, and police documents may display regular paterns of assault or drunk and disorderly behaviour. Even prison files may exhibit evidence of regular monthly episodes of bizarre behaviour occurring while in custody. All such information is valuable in building up positive evidence that the woman has symptoms at menstruation with normal behaviour at other times.

Other diagnostic pointers worth bearing in mind are the frequency with which the onset of PMS, and the occasions of increased severity, occur at times of upheaval of the menstrual hormones. These times include puberty, after pregnancy, during or after stopping the pill, after a spell of amenorrhea such as occurs in anorexia nervosa, and following sterilization. Women with PMS usually have normal, pain-free and regular menstruation, and never experience the spasms of lower abdominal colicky pains so typical of spasmodic dysmenorrhea.

Women with PMS are usually the ones who develop side effects on the pill, complaining that it causes headaches, depression or weight gain. They change their brand of pill and finally resort to some other contraceptive method. There is a high incidence of about nine women in every ten who develop PMS after certain complications associated with pregnancy. These include pre-eclampsia severe enough to require hospital admission in the antenatal period, or postnatal depression severe enough to need antidepressant treatment in the puerperium. There may also be a history of a threatened miscarriage in the early months with a successful outcome of pregnancy.

Body Chemistry

During the premenstruum, women with PMS experience a rise in glucose tolerance which results in food cravings and binges. The frequent weight gain and bloatedness in the premenstruum brings with it a desire to diet, so causing problems of intermittent feasting and famine. When PMS sufferers go too long without food, their blood glucose level reaches baseline and there is a compensating spurt of adrenalin to release glucose from the body's store. It is this sudden release of adrenalin which is reponsible for many of the premenstrual symptoms such as panic attacks, explosive outbursts, uncontrollable aggression and migraine. After all, adrenalin is recognized as the hormone of fear, fight and flight. Careful enquiry will elicit the fact that most instances of baby battering and assault occur after a long food gap (five hours in the day or thirteen hours overnight). The mother who misses breakfast is most likely to be irritable at lunchtime, and the housewife who forgets her midday meal will be aggressive when her husband returns from work in the evening.

Alcohol tolerance varies over the menstrual cycle and those with PMS may find that during the premenstruum they are unable to tolerate their normal alcohol intake without signs of intoxication. The problem is increased by their urges to take alcohol at this time to overcome their premenstrual depression and lethargy. Thus during the premenstruum, at a time of lowered self-discipline, lowered self-control, alcohol urges and increased tendency to intoxication, is it any wonder that charges of drunk and disorderly occur with such frequency on the woman's charge sheets? Yet these same women may have no difficulty in totally abstaining from alcohol at other times of the menstrual cycle.

Conclusion

One in ten of all menstruating women are estimated to suffer from PMS severe enough to require treatment. Diagnosis is simple, but the responsibility of referring possible sufferers to their general practitioner frequently rests with health visitors, and they should not fail in this task.

APPENDIX II

PMS Support Groups and Clinics in the U.S.A. (1983)

Any such listing cannot be up-to-date and comprehensive because new groups are being created all the time. Updated information may be available from the publisher of this book. The list below merely gives some idea of the progress.

These addresses and related information are supplied as a service to the reader but in no way constitute a recommendation or endorsement of any particular group or service. The author and publishers cannot be held liable for any results from self-treatment or treatment at any of these facilities.

THE NATIONAL PMS SOCIETY

P.O. Box 11467   Lindsay Burton Leckie
Durham, NC 27703   Michele Council
(919) 489-6577/6578

The National PMS Society is a non-profit, all volunteer, educational and support network consisting of 91 affiliated groups throughout the country. Their goals are to educate the medical and lay community in the identification and the treatment of PMS, to promote among the general public an awareness of the existence of PMS, and to assist women by offering emotional support and up-dated information. This information is available through the Society's own literature and newsletters as well as other literature on PMS. Other activities include walk-in counseling, telephone hotlines, public meetings, workshops and seminars. Future goals are to raise money for PMS research. Approved by Dr. Katharina Dalton.

PMS ACTION, INC.
P.O. Box 9236   Virginia Cassara
Madison, WI 53715
(608) 274-6688

PMS Action is a non-profit corporation founded in May, 1980, as the first organization committed to increasing awareness about PMS. The organization's goals are to further the recognition of PMS as a physiological disorder. This is done by educating health, social service professionals and laypersons about PMS and its treatment.

PMS SUPPORT AND EDUCATION CENTER

1324 Westwood Blvd.   Jill Kaufman
Los Angeles, CA 90024   Joyce Lederer
(213) 477-0938   Marilyn Brown
                                          Norma Freeman

The PMS Support and Education Center is a non-profit support and educational program to inform women how to be medical consumers and to be aware of medical advances—specifically in childbirth, postnatal problems and premenstrual issues. Treatment programs consist of psychological and dietary therapy and medical referrals. Literature is available through the Center, and workshops and seminars are held.
Approved by Dr. Katharina Dalton.

FAMILY AND TEEN HEALTH SERVICES/ PMS PROGRAM

Greene County Memorial Hospital   Bonita Roche
Bonar & 7th Ave.
Waynesburg, PA 15370
(412) 627-3865/3101

This is a non-profit, hospital-based health care facility that serves as a premenstrual syndrome treatment, community education and information center. Information is available through literature, workshops and seminars.
Approved by Dr. Katharina Dalton.

PMS CENTER OF ORANGE COUNTY

(MacArthur Medical Center)   Charles B. Bartell, M.D.
18021 Sky Park — Suite H   Barbara Jernigan
Irvine, CA 92714   Brenda Moyes
(714) 261-7372/6390

PMS Center of Orange County is a complete medical center
that aims to educate and treat women with PMS through the
services of physicians, psychiatrists, nurse consultants, and a
nutritionist. Approved by Dr. Katharina Dalton.

FRANK WM. VARESE, M.D.

24953 Paseo de Valencia #7C
Laguna Hills, CA 92653
(714) 837-1510/1711

Dr. Varese is a family practitioner who diagnoses and treats
PMS. He was trained and certified in London, England by Dr.
Katharina Dalton.

PMS TREATMENT CENTER

735 W. Duarte Rd., #206   Holly Anderson
Arcadia, CA 91006   Alvin L. Hensel, M.D.
(213) 447-0679/0670

The PMS Treatment Center is a professional organization
whose main goals are to effectively treat women with PMS and
to raise the consciousness of the public regarding this disease.
Seminars are conducted and booklets are available through the
Center on PMS and natural progesterone therapy.

PMS CENTER
9201 Sunset Blvd., #906   Lloyd Byron Greig, M.D.
Los Angeles, CA 90069
(213) 276-1151/1152

The PMS Center is a professional, physician directed organization for the evaluation and treatment of PMS.

PMS INSTITUTE
4541 N. 7th St.   Marshall Smith, M.D., Ph.D.
Phoenix, AZ   Celia Halas, Ph.D.
(602) 279-2233   Pat Yorke

The PMS Institute is a professional organization specializing in the evaluation and treatment of PMS with collection of data for research. It provides patients with a library of pertinent material including books, magazine articles and tapes.

VANDERBILT UNIVERSITY PMS PROGRAM
Dept of OB/GYN   Judy Belsito, MSSW
Vanderbilt Medical Center   Dr. Stephen Entman
Nashville, TN 37232   Dr. Wayne Maxson
(615) 322-3447   Sue Jones, Ms. R.N.

This program is an academic study group, non-profit and professional. Their goals are to conduct research study regarding PMS and the efficacy of progesterone therapy. Although they are primarily research oriented, treatment is available for women with severe PMS.

PMS PROGRAM, INC.
40 Salem St.   Karen Schlotman
Lynnfield, MA 01701
(617) 245-9585

800 Eastowne Dr.   Judy Coons, R.N.
Chapel Hill, NC
(919) 493-5427

2656 S. Loop West   Cindy Dear, R.N.
Houston, TX
(713)661-6644

The PMS Program is comprised of professional medical offices established for the purpose of evaluating and treating women who suffer from premenstrual syndrome, and to carry out research in regard to this disorder.

PMS RELIEF
P.O. Box 10   Gillian Ford
Newcastle, CA 59658
(916) 888-7677

PMS Relief is basically a counseling and referral organization whose goal is to inform women about PMS. Literature is distributed and seminars are held.

PMS SUPPORT GROUP, INC.
P.O. Box 600   Sandy Bammer
64 Rockridge
Woodacre, CA 94973
(415) 488-4052

A professional (non-profit pending) information, referral and support group whose goals are to educate women, their families and friends, the community and employers about PMS. Information includes literature, workshops and seminars.

PMS RESEARCH FOUNDATION
P.O. Box 14574   Lee Horner
Las Vegas, NV 89114
(702) 369-9248

The PMS Research Foundation is aimed at collecting and disseminating information to educate women about PMS. Aside from their continuous library and field research, the Foundation also provides support groups and workshops on local and international levels, literature and an interchange of information with individuals and organizations concerned with the control of PMS. A local medical referral service and a PMS Speakers Bureau are also available.

PMS COMMUNITY AWARENESS
1914 Chandler Lane   Laurie Woodall
Columbus, IN 47203
(812) 372-5340

This group has been active since November 1982 and is in the process of becoming a non-profit organization. The basic goals of PMS Community Awareness is to inform the public and refer PMS sufferers to appropriate doctors. Activities include monthly meetings, support groups and public speakers.

UTAH PMS CENTER
667 East 100 South, Suite 300   Patty Cannon, Director
Salt Lake City, UT 84102   Co-founder,
(801) 322-5100   National PMS Society
                                      William R. Keye, M.D.
                                  Chairman, Advisory Board

This group is engaged in research, education, diagnosis, medical treatment, and support for women suffering from premenstrual syndrome and its related problems. Their goals are to explore and implement the medical treatment of premenstrual syndrome, and to collect and report data to other practitioners.

Index

Index

Use This Handy Order Form
for Your *SPECIAL DISCOUNT*
on Hunter House
Family & Health Books

ONCE A MONTH by Katharina Dalton, M.D.

A clear, myth free book about the premenstrual syndrome, its effects, and complete treatment. The SECOND EDITION has been fully updated with important new information including PMS: LEGAL & DIAGNOSTIC GUIDE-LINES and PMS GROUPS: A DIRECTORY.

2nd Revised Edition   256pp   Soft Cover $6.95
1st Edition   224pp   Soft Cover $4.95

PATTERNS: The Fertility Awareness Book by Barbara Kass-Annese, R.N., N.P., & Hal C. Danzer, M.D.

A clearly illustrated, easy-to-read book that combines accurate information about reproduction with the concepts of Fertility Awareness and Natural Family Planning. Designed and written by experts in the field of reproduction and health care to fill a real educational need.

2nd Revised Edition   112pp   Soft Cover $9.95
1st Edition   112pp   Soft Cover $7.95

EXCLUSIVELY FEMALE: A Nutrition Guide for Better Menstrual Health by Linda Ojeda

This book explores menstrual problems that may result from nutritional deficiencies. With proper nutrition, these symptoms can be minimized if not totally relieved. "Every woman should read and apply the principles of this book." — *Kurt W. Donsbach, Ph.D.*

Revised Edition   128pp   Soft Cover $4.50

DRINKING PROBLEMS = FAMILY PROBLEMS by Marie-Louise Meyer, R.N.

This book provides guidelines for dealing with the problem drinker at home, in the family, at work, and at play. How to help, how to cope, and how — and when — to release: it's all examined here. A clear discussion on the choices that must be made.

1st Edition   256pp   Hard Cover $12.95

See over for ordering & discounts

Cut Here

DISCOUNT POLICY

20% DISCOUNT on orders of **$20.** or more —
A savings of at least **$4.**

25% DISCOUNT on orders of **$50.** or more —
A savings of at least **$12.50.**

30% DISCOUNT on orders of **$250.** or more —
A savings of at least **$75.**

Add postage and handling at $1.50 for one book and $0.50 for every additional book. Please allow 6 to 8 weeks for delivery.

Name_____

Street/Number_____

City/State _____ Zip_____

SEND ME:

ONCE A MONTH (2nd Ed.) .... _____ @ $ 6.95 _____

ONCE A MONTH (1st Ed.) .... _____ @ $ 4.95 _____

PATTERNS (2nd Ed.) .... _____ @ $ 9.95 _____

PATTERNS (1st Ed.) .... _____ @ $ 7.95 _____

EXCLUSIVELY FEMALE .... _____ @ $ 4.50 _____

DRINKING PROBLEMS .... _____ @ $12.95 _____

TOTAL _____

DISCOUNT AT _____%   **LESS** $(_____)

TOTAL COST OF BOOKS $_____

Shipping & Handling $_____

California Residents add Sales Tax $_____

TOTAL AMOUNT ENCLOSED $_____

☐ Cash   ☐ Check   ☐ Money Order

☐ Check here to receive our catalog of books

Please complete and mail to:
HUNTER HOUSE INC., PUBLISHERS
PO Box 1302, Claremont, CA 91711, USA

If you don't use this offer — give it to a friend!

Use This Handy Order Form
for Your *SPECIAL DISCOUNT*
on Hunter House
Family & Health Books

ONCE A MONTH by Katharina Dalton, M.D.

A clear, myth free book about the premenstrual syndrome, its effects, and complete treatment. The SECOND EDITION has been fully updated with important new information including PMS: LEGAL & DIAGNOSTIC GUIDE-LINES and PMS GROUPS: A DIRECTORY.

2nd Revised Edition   256pp   Soft Cover $6.95
1st Edition   224pp   Soft Cover $4.95

PATTERNS: The Fertility Awareness Book by Barbara Kass-Annese, R.N., N.P., & Hal C. Danzer, M.D.

A clearly illustrated, easy-to-read book that combines accurate information about reproduction with the concepts of Fertility Awareness and Natural Family Planning. Designed and written by experts in the field of reproduction and health care to fill a real educational need.

2nd Revised Edition   112pp   Soft Cover $9.95
1st Edition   112pp   Soft Cover $7.95

EXCLUSIVELY FEMALE: A Nutrition Guide for Better Menstrual Health by Linda Ojeda

This book explores menstrual problems that may result from nutritional deficiencies. With proper nutrition, these symptoms can be minimized if not totally relieved. "Every woman should read and apply the principles of this book." — *Kurt W. Donsbach, Ph.D.*

Revised Edition   128pp   Soft Cover $4.50

DRINKING PROBLEMS = FAMILY PROBLEMS by Marie-Louise Meyer, R.N.

This book provides guidelines for dealing with the problem drinker at home, in the family, at work, and at play. How to help, how to cope, and how — and when — to release: it's all examined here. A clear discussion on the choices that must be made.

1st Edition   256pp   Hard Cover $12.95

See over for ordering & discounts

Cut Here